P9-CRK-144

PN Mental Health Nursing
Review Module Edition 8.0

Contributors

Audrey Knippa, MS, MPH, RN, CNE
Nursing Education Coordinator and
  Content Project Leader

Sheryl Sommer, PhD, MSN, RN, CNE
Director, Nursing Curriculum and
  Education Services

Brenda Ball, MEd, BSN, RN
Nursing Education Specialist

Lois Churchill, MN, RN
Nursing Education Specialist

Carrie B. Elkins, DHSc, MSN, PHCNS, BC
Nursing Education Specialist

Mary Jane Janowski, MA, BSN, RN
Nursing Resource Specialist

Sharon R. Redding, EdD, RN, CNE
Nursing Education Specialist

Karin Roberts, PhD, MSN, RN, CNE
Nursing Education Coordinator

Mendy G. Wright, DNP, MSN, RN
Nursing Education Specialist

Chris Crawford, BS Journalism
Product Developer and Editorial Project Leader

Derek Prater, MS Journalism
Lead Product Developer

Johanna Barnes, BA Journalism
Product Developer

Joey Berlin, BS Journalism
Product Developer

Hilary E. Groninger, BS Journalism
Product Developer

Megan E. Herre, BS Journalism
Product Developer

Amanda Lehman, BA English
Product Developer

Spring Lenox, BS Journalism
Product Developer

Robin Nelson, BA English
Product Developer

Joanna Shindler, BA Journalism
Product Developer

Morgan Smith, BS Journalism
Media Developer

Brant L. Stacy, BS Journalism, BA English
Product Developer

Mandy Tallmadge, BS Communication
Product Developer

Karen D. Wood, BS Journalism
Product Developer

Katherine Wood-Raclin, BA English, Mass
Communications
Product Developer

Consultants

Christina D. Brazier, MSN, RN

Phyllis M. Jacobs, MSN, RN

Linda Turchin, MSN, RN, CNE

INTELLECTUAL PROPERTY NOTICE

IMPORTANT NOTICE TO THE READER

USER'S GUIDE

Welcome to the Assessment Technologies Institute® PN Mental Health Nursing Review Module Edition 8.0. The mission of ATI's Content Mastery Series® review modules is to provide user-friendly compendiums of nursing knowledge that will:

- Help you locate important information quickly.

- Assist in your remediation efforts.

- Provide exercises for applying your nursing knowledge.

- Facilitate your entry into the nursing profession as a newly licensed PN.

Organization

This review module is organized into units covering foundations for mental health nursing, traditional nonpharmacological therapies, psychobiologic disorders, psychopharmacological therapies, special populations, and psychiatric emergencies. Chapters within these units conform to one of four organizing principles for presenting the content:

- Basic concepts

- Procedures (diagnostic and therapeutic)

- Systems disorders

- Medications

Basic concepts chapters begin with an overview describing the central concept and its relevance to nursing. Subordinate themes are in outline form to demonstrate relationships and present the information in a clear, succinct manner.

Procedures chapters include an overview describing the procedure(s) covered in the chapter. These chapters will provide you with nursing knowledge relevant to each procedure, including indications, interpretations of findings, client outcomes, nursing actions, and complications.

Systems disorders chapters include an overview describing the disorder. These chapters cover data collection, including risk factors, subjective data, and objective data, and collaborative care, including nursing care, medications, interdisciplinary care, therapeutic procedures, and client outcomes.

Medications chapters include an overview describing a disorder, group of disorders or specific medication classifications. Sections within the chapters will focus on a prototype or prototype medications. These sections include information about how the medication works, its therapeutic uses, and routes of administration. Next, you will find information about complications, contraindications, and medication and food interactions, as well as nursing interventions and client education to help prevent and/or manage these issues. Finally, the chapter includes information on nursing administration of the medication and evaluation of the medication's effectiveness.

Application Exercises

At the end of each chapter there are questions you can use to practice applying your knowledge. The Application Exercises include both NCLEX-style questions, such as multiple-choice and multiple-select items, and questions that ask you to apply your knowledge in other formats, such as short-answer and matching items. After completing the Application Exercises, go to the Application Exercise Answer Key to check your answers and rationales for correct and incorrect answers.

NCLEX® Connections

To prepare for the NCLEX-PN, it is important for you to understand how the content in this review module is connected to the NCLEX-PN test plan. You can find information on the detailed test plan at the National Council of State Boards of Nursing's Web site: https://www.ncsbn.org/. When reviewing content in this review module, regularly ask yourself, "How does this content fit into the test plan, and what types of questions related to this content should I expect?"

To help you in this process, we've included NCLEX Connections at the beginning of each unit and with each question in the Application Exercises Answer Keys. The NCLEX Connections at the beginning of each unit will point out areas of the detailed test plan that relate to the content within that unit. The NCLEX Connections attached to the Application Exercises Answer Keys will demonstrate how each exercise fits within the detailed content outline.

These NCLEX Connections will help you understand how the detailed content outline is organized, starting with major client needs categories and subcategories and followed by related content areas and tasks. The major client needs categories are:

- Safe and Effective Care Environment
  - Management of Care
  - Safety and Infection Control
- Health Promotion and Maintenance
- Psychosocial Integrity
- Physiological Integrity
  - Basic Care and Comfort
  - Pharmacological Therapies
  - Reduction of Risk Potential
  - Physiological Adaptation

An NCLEX Connection might, for example, alert you that content within a unit is related to:

- Psychosocial Integrity
  - Behavioral Management
    - Explore cause of client behavior.

Icons

Throughout the review module you will see icons that will draw your attention to particular areas. Keep an eye out for these icons:

 This icon indicates an Overview, or introduction, to a particular subject matter. Descriptions and categories will typically be found in an Overview.

 This icon indicates Application Exercises and Application Exercises Answer Keys.

 This icon indicates NCLEX connections.

 This icon indicates gerontological content. When you see this icon, take note of information that is specific to aging or the care of older adult clients.

 This icon indicates content related to safety. When you see this icon, take note of safety concerns or steps that nurses can take to ensure client safety and a safe environment.

 This icon indicates that a media supplement, such as a graphic, an animation, or a video, is available. If you have an electronic copy of the review module, this icon will appear alongside clickable links to media supplements. If you have a hardcopy version of the review module, visit www.atitesting.com for details on how to access these features.

Feedback

ATI welcomes feedback regarding this review module. Please provide comments to: comments@atitesting.com.

Table of Contents

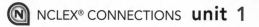

UNIT 1: FOUNDATIONS FOR MENTAL HEALTH NURSING

- Basic Mental Health Nursing Concepts

- Legal and Ethical Issues

- Effective Communication

- Anxiety and Defense Mechanisms

- Creating and Maintaining a Therapeutic and Safe Environment

---

NCLEX® CONNECTIONS

When reviewing the chapters in this section, keep in mind the relevant sections of the NCLEX® outline, in particular:

CLIENT NEEDS: MANAGEMENT OF CARE

Relevant topics/tasks include:
- Advocacy
  - Advocate for client rights or needs.
- Client Rights
  - Intervene if client rights are violated.
- Ethical Practice
  - Identify ethical issues affecting staff or client.

CLIENT NEEDS: SAFETY AND INFECTION CONTROL

Relevant topics/tasks include:
- Accident/Error/Injury Prevention
  - Recognize what factors related to mental status may contribute to the client potential for accident or injury.
- Restraints and Safety Devices
  - Implement least restrictive restraints for seclusion.

CLIENT NEEDS: PSYCHOSOCIAL INTEGRITY

Relevant topics/tasks include:
- Coping Mechanisms
  - Identify client use of effective and ineffective coping mechanisms.
- Therapeutic Communication
  - Use therapeutic communication techniques with client.
- Therapeutic Environment
  - Contribute to maintaining a safe and supportive environment for client.

UNIT 1	FOUNDATIONS FOR MENTAL HEALTH NURSING
Chapter 1	Basic Mental Health Nursing Concepts

 Overview

- Provision of care to clients in mental health settings is based on standards of care set by the American Nurses Association, the American Psychiatric Nurses Association, and the International Society of Psychiatric-Mental Health Nurses. Foundational to this care is the use of the nursing process.

- Mental health nurses should use the nursing process, as well as a holistic approach (biological, social, psychological, spiritual aspects) to care for clients in mental health settings.

- Various methods should be used to identify factors that impact the mental well-being of clients. These methods include observation, interviewing, physical examination, and collaboration.

Data Collection

- Data collection is ongoing and involves monitoring the status of the client with each encounter.

- Psychosocial History

  o Perception of own health, beliefs about illness and wellness

  o Activity and leisure activities (how the client passes time)

  o Use and possible abuse of substances

  o Stress level and coping abilities (usual coping strategies, support systems)

  o Cultural beliefs and practices

  o Spiritual beliefs

- The Mental Status Examination (MSE)

(M) **View Media Supplement:** Mental Status Examination (Video)

- o Level of consciousness is described using the following terms, and observed behavior should be included in documentation:
  - Alert
    - □ Clients are responsive and able to fully respond by opening their eyes and attending to a normal tone of voice and speech. They answer questions spontaneously and appropriately.
  - Lethargy
    - □ Clients are able to open their eyes and respond but are drowsy and fall asleep readily.
  - Obtundation
    - □ Clients need to be lightly shaken to elicit a response, but they may be confused and slow to respond.
  - Stupor
    - □ Clients require painful stimuli (pinching a tendon, rubbing the sternum) to elicit a brief response. They may not be able to respond verbally.
  - Coma
    - □ No response can be achieved from repeated painful stimuli.
      - ‣ Abnormal posturing in the client who is comatose
      - ‣ Decorticate rigidity – Flexion and internal rotation of upper-extremity joints and legs
      - ‣ Decerebrate rigidity – Neck and elbow extension and wrist and finger flexion
- o Physical appearance
  - Examination includes evaluation of client's personal hygiene, grooming, and clothing choice. Expected findings with regard to evaluation are that the client is well-kept, clean, and dressed appropriately for the given environment.
- o Behavior
  - Examination includes observation of voluntary and involuntary body movements, and eye contact.
    - □ Mood – Provides information about the emotion that the client is feeling
    - □ Affect – An objective expression of mood, such as a flat affect or a lack of facial expression
- o Cognitive and intellectual abilities
  - Determine the client's orientation to time, person, and place.
  - Evaluate the client's memory, both recent and remote.
    - □ Recent – Ask the client to repeat a series of numbers or a list of objects.
    - □ Remote – Ask the client to state a fact that is verifiable, such as his birth date or his mother's maiden name.

- Evaluate the client's level of knowledge. For example, ask him what he knows about his current illness or hospitalization.

- Evaluate the client's ability to calculate. (Can the client count backwards from 100 in multiples of 7?)

- Evaluate the client's ability to think abstractly. (Can the client interpret a cliché, such as, "A bird in the hand is worth two in the bush."?) The ability to interpret this demonstrates a higher level thought process.

- Ask the questions to determine the client's perception of her illness.

- Evaluate the client's judgment based on his answer to a hypothetical question. (How would the client answer the question, "What would you do if there were a fire in your room?") The response to the question should be logical.

- Evaluate the client's rate and volume of speech, as well as the quality of his language. His speech should be articulate and his responses meaningful and appropriate.

- Standardized Screening Tools

  - Mini-Mental State Examination (MMSE)

    - This examination is used to objectively evaluate a client's cognitive status by determining the following:

      - Orientation to time and place

      - Attention span and ability to calculate by counting backwards in multiples of seven

      - Registration and recalling of objects

      - Language, including naming of objects, following commands, and ability to write

  - Glasgow Coma Scale

    - This examination is used to obtain baseline data about a client's level of consciousness and for ongoing evaluation of the client.

    - Eye, verbal, and motor response is evaluated, and a number value based on that response is assigned. The highest value possible is 15, which indicates that the client is awake and responding appropriately. A score of 3 indicates that the client is in a coma.

Considerations Across the Lifespan

- Children and Adolescents

  - Evaluate the client's temperament, social and environmental factors, cultural and religious concerns, and developmental level.

  - Mentally healthy children and adolescents should trust others, view the world as safe, accurately interpret their environments, master developmental tasks, and use appropriate coping skills.

- o Children and adolescents experience some of the same mental health problems as adults.

- o Mental health and developmental disorders are not always easily diagnosed, and treatment interventions may be delayed or inadequate. Factors contributing to this include:

    - Lack of the ability or necessary skills to describe what is happening

    - A wide variation of "normal" behavior, especially in different developmental stages

- o Observe this age group for mood, anxiety, developmental, behavioral, and eating disorders. A risk of suicide should also be considered.

- • The Older Adult

    - o In addition to the aforementioned data to be collected, the nurse should evaluate older adult clients for the following factors:

        - Functional ability, such as the ability to get up out of a chair

        - Economic and social status

        - Environmental factors, such as stairways in the home, that may affect the client's well-being and lifestyle

    - o Standardized assessment tools that are specific to the older adult population, include:

        - Geriatric Depression Scale (short form)

        - Michigan Alcoholism Screening Test – Geriatric Version

        - MMSE

        - Pain assessments, including visual analogue scales, Wong-Baker FACES Pain Rating Scale, the McGill Pain Questionnaire (MPQ), and the Pain Assessment in Advanced Dementia (PAINAD) scale

- • Use the following strategies when collecting data from all clients:

    - o Use a private, quiet space with adequate lighting to accommodate for impaired vision and hearing.

    - o Make an introduction and determine the client's name preference.

    - o Stand or sit at the client's level to conduct the interview, rather than standing over a client who is bed bound or sitting in a chair.

    - o Respect the client's personal space if he does not wish to be touched, but use touch to communicate caring as appropriate.

    - o Be sure to include questions relating to difficulty sleeping, incontinence, falls or other injuries, depression, dizziness, and loss of energy.

    - o Include the family and significant others as appropriate.

    - o Take a detailed medication history.

    - o Following the interview, summarize and ask for feedback from the client.

Mental Health Diagnoses

- The Diagnostic and Statistical Manual of Mental Disorders, 4th Edition, text revision (DSM-IV-TR), published by the American Psychiatric Association, is used as a diagnostic tool to identify medical diagnoses. It is used by mental health professionals for clients who have mental health disorders.

- Nurses use the DSM-IV-TR in the mental health setting to identify diagnoses and diagnostic criteria to guide data collection, and to plan, implement, and evaluate care.

- Multiaxial System – The DSM-IV-TR uses a multiaxial system to assess clients in the mental health setting. It assesses for abnormal behavior, comorbid medical conditions, conditions within the environment, and level of functioning.

  o Axis I – All mental health diagnosis except for those found in Axis II

  o Axis II – Any personality disorder diagnosis and mental retardation

  o Axis III – Any general medical diagnosis, such as asthma

  o Axis IV – Pertinent psychosocial problems and problems that may affect diagnosis, treatment, and prognosis of mental disorders, such as poor family support

  o Axis V – Global assessment of functioning (GAF) – An assessment of present and past-year functioning that rates the client's level of functioning in the areas of work performance, social abilities, and psychological ability on a scale of 1 to 100.

    ▪ Scores of 80 to 100 generally indicate normal or near-normal function.

    ▪ Scores of 60 to 80 indicate moderate problems.

    ▪ Scores 40 and below indicate serious mental disability and/or functioning impairments.

    ▪ Present and past-year GAF scores are compared to track the client's level of functioning. For example, a GAF of 50/80 indicates that the client presently has a GAF score of 50, with a previous score of 80 in the past year.

Therapeutic Strategies in the Mental Health Setting

MENTAL HEALTH NURSING INTERVENTIONS	
Counseling	• Use therapeutic communication skills. • Assist with problem solving. • Identify a crisis intervention. • Assist with stress management.
Milieu therapy	• Orient clients to the physical setting. • Identify rules and boundaries of the setting. • Ensure a safe environment for clients. • Assist clients to participate in appropriate activities.
Promotion of self-care activities	• Offer assistance with self-care tasks. • Allow time for the client to complete self-care tasks. • Set incentives to promote client self-care.
Psychobiological interventions	• Administer prescribed medications. • Reinforce teaching to the client/family. • Monitor for side effects and effectiveness of therapy.
Cognitive and behavioral therapies	• Modeling • Operant conditioning • Systematic desensitization
Health teaching	• Encourage the development of social and coping skills.
Health promotion and health maintenance	• Assist clients with cessation of smoking. • Monitor other health conditions.

Ⓐ APPLICATION EXERCISES

1. While performing a mental status examination on a client, the nurse notices that the client's facial expression constantly conveys anger. The nurse should document this information as part of the client's

    A. orientation.

    B. appearance.

    C. affect.

    D. consciousness.

2. During a mental status examination, a client who is hospitalized states that she is undergoing treatment "to learn how to become a doctor." The nurse should record this information as

    A. poor perception of illness.

    B. decreased level of knowledge.

    C. decreased judgment.

    D. poor remote memory.

3. Which of the following are examples of subjective data collection? (Select all that apply.)

    _____ Client's speech is slow and soft

    _____ Client states he has no reason to live

    _____ Client is able to recall three numbers

    _____ Client meditates for relaxation

    _____ Client states that he drinks three beers a day

4. A nurse is caring for a client diagnosed with schizophrenia, diabetes mellitus, major depressive disorder, and antisocial personality disorder. Which of the following diagnoses should the nurse expect to find included on Axis II of this client's DSM-IV-TR axis diagnoses?

    A. Schizophrenia

    B. Diabetes mellitus

    C. Major depressive disorder

    D. Antisocial personality disorder

5. A client is admitted to an acute care mental health facility. The following medical diagnoses and psychosocial information are available at the time of admission: hypertension, mild mental retardation, and dysthymic disorder. The client's highest level of functioning from a global assessment of functioning (GAF) performed a year ago was 50. Today, the highest level of functioning on the same scale is 20. The client has been taking other clients' possessions at the group home. How should the nurse enter all of this information into the multiaxial system of the DSM-IV-TR?

(A) APPLICATION EXERCISES ANSWER KEY

1. While performing a mental status examination on a client, the nurse notices that the client's facial expression constantly conveys anger. The nurse should document this information as part of the client's

    A. orientation.

    B. appearance.

    C. affect.

    D. consciousness.

    The nurse should describe this client's facial expression as a component of his affect, not as his orientation, appearance, or consciousness.

 NCLEX® Connection: Psychosocial Integrity, Mental Health Concepts

2. During a mental status examination, a client who is hospitalized states that she is undergoing treatment "to learn how to become a doctor." The nurse should record this information as

    A. poor perception of illness.

    B. decreased level of knowledge.

    C. decreased judgment.

    D. poor remote memory.

    The nurse's objective collection of data about the client's insight reflects the client's lack of understanding or perception of her current situation and medical status. Knowledge, judgment, and memory are other objective cognitive data that do not reflect the client's understanding of her responsibility for, or analysis of, her current situation.

 NCLEX® Connection: Psychosocial Integrity, Mental Health Concepts

3. Which of the following are examples of subjective data collection? (Select all that apply.)

    _____ Client's speech is slow and soft

    __X__ **Client states he has no reason to live**

    _____ Client is able to recall three numbers

    _____ Client meditates for relaxation

    __X__ **Client states that he drinks three beers a day**

    Subjective data include psychosocial information about the client's thoughts, actions, and feelings that can only be described by the client. Objective data are based on observable or verifiable facts.

 NCLEX® Connection: Psychosocial Integrity, Mental Health Concepts

4. A nurse is caring for a client diagnosed with schizophrenia, diabetes mellitus, major depressive disorder, and antisocial personality disorder. Which of the following diagnoses should the nurse expect to find included on Axis II of this client's DSM-IV-TR axis diagnoses?

    A. Schizophrenia

    B. Diabetes mellitus

    C. Major depressive disorder

    D. Antisocial personality disorder

    Personality disorders and mental retardation are included on Axis II. Schizophrenia and major depressive disorder are found on Axis I. Diabetes mellitus and other general medical disorders are found on Axis III.

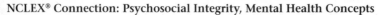 NCLEX® Connection: Psychosocial Integrity, Mental Health Concepts

5. A client is admitted to an acute care mental health facility. The following medical diagnoses and psychosocial information are available at the time of admission: hypertension, mild mental retardation, and dysthymic disorder. The client's highest level of functioning from a global assessment of functioning (GAF) performed a year ago was 50. Today, the highest level of functioning on the same scale is 20. The client has been taking other clients' possessions at the group home. How should the nurse enter all of this information into the multiaxial system of the DSM-IV-TR?

    Axis I: Dysthymic disorder

    Axis II: Mild mental retardation

    Axis III: Hypertension

    Axis IV: Has been taking other clients' possessions at group home

    Axis V: GAF 20/50

    Axis I includes most mental health clinical disorders, except those placed on Axis II. Axis II disorders include personality disorders and mental retardation. Axis III includes general medical disorders and problems. Axis IV includes pertinent psychosocial information or problems with living conditions. Axis V includes GAF for the present observation and a previous evaluation within 1 year of the present observation.

NCLEX® Connection: Psychosocial Integrity, Mental Health Concepts

UNIT 1	FOUNDATIONS FOR MENTAL HEALTH NURSING
Chapter 2	Legal and Ethical Issues

Overview

- A nurse who works in the mental health setting is responsible for practicing ethically, competently, safely, and in a manner consistent with all local, state, and federal laws.

- Nurses must have an understanding of ethical principles and how they apply when providing care for clients in mental health settings.

- Nurses are responsible for understanding and protecting client rights.

Legal Rights of Clients in the Mental Health Setting

- Clients who have been diagnosed and/or hospitalized with a mental health disorder are guaranteed the same civil rights as any other citizen. These include:

  o The right to humane treatment and care, such as medical and dental care

  o The right to vote in national, state, and local government elections

  o The right to due process of law, including the right to press legal charges against another person

- Clients also have various specific rights, including:

  o Informed consent and the right to refuse treatment

  o Confidentiality

  o A written plan of care/treatment that includes discharge follow-up, as well as participation in the care plan and review of that plan

  o Communication with persons outside the mental health facility, including family members, attorneys, and other health care professionals

  o Provision of adequate interpretive services if needed

  o Care provided with respect, dignity, and without discrimination

  o Freedom from harm related to physical or pharmacologic restraint, seclusion, and any physical or mental abuse or neglect

  o Provision of care with the least restrictive interventions necessary to meet the client's needs without allowing him to be a threat to himself or others

- Some legal issues regarding health care may be decided in court using a specialized civil category called a tort. A tort is a wrongful act or injury committed by an entity or person against another person or another person's property. Torts can be used to decide liability issues, as well as intentional issues that may involve criminal penalties, such as abuse of a client.

- State laws can vary greatly. The nurse must be aware of specific laws regarding client care within the state or states in which the nurse practices.

Ethical Issues for Clients in the Mental Health Setting

- In comparison to laws, statutes, and regulations enacted by local, state, or federal government, ethical issues are philosophical ideas regarding right and wrong.

- Nurses are frequently confronted with ethical dilemmas regarding client care (bioethical issues).

- Since ethics are philosophical and involve values and morals, there is frequently no clear-cut simple resolution to an ethical dilemma.

- Ethical principles must be used to decide ethical issues. These include:

ETHICAL PRINCIPLE	DEFINITION	EXAMPLE
Beneficence	This relates to the quality of doing good and can be described as charity.	A nurse helps a newly admitted client who has psychosis feel safe in the environment of the mental health facility.
Autonomy	This refers to the client's right to make his own decisions, but the client must accept the consequences of those decisions. The client must also respect the decisions of others.	Rather than giving advice to a client who has difficulty making decisions, a nurse helps the client explore all alternatives, arrive at a choice, and understand the consequences of the various decisions.
Justice	This is defined as fair and equal treatment for all.	During a treatment team meeting, a nurse leads a discussion regarding whether or not two clients who broke the same facility rule were treated equally.
Fidelity	This relates to loyalty and faithfulness to the client and to one's duty.	A client asks a nurse to be present when she talks to her mother for the first time in a year. The nurse remains with the client during this interaction.
Veracity	This refers to being honest when dealing with a client.	A client states, "You and that other staff member were talking about me, weren't you?" The nurse truthfully replies, "We were discussing ways to help you relate to the other clients in a more positive way."

Confidentiality

- The client's right to privacy is protected by the Health Insurance Portability and Accountability Act (HIPAA) of 2003.

- It is important to gain an understanding of the federal law and of various state laws as they relate to confidentiality in specific health care facilities.

- Information about the client, verbal and in writing, must only be shared with those who are responsible for implementing the client's treatment plan.

- Information may be shared with other persons not involved in the client treatment plan by client consent only.

- Specific mental health issues include disclosing HIV status, the duty to warn and protect third parties, and the reporting of child and elder abuse.

Resources for Solving Ethical Client Issues

- Code of Ethics for Nurses (http://nursingworld.org/)

- Patient Care Partnership (http://www.aha.org/)

- The nurse practice act of a specific state

- Legal advice from attorneys

- Facility policies

- Other members of the health care team, including facility bioethics committee (if available)

- Members of the clergy and other spiritual or ethical counselors

Types of Commitment to a Mental Health Facility

- Voluntary commitment – The client or client's guardian chooses commitment to a mental health facility in order to obtain treatment. A voluntarily committed client has the right to apply for release at any time. This client is considered competent, and so has the right to refuse medication and treatment.

- Involuntary (civil) commitment – The client enters the mental health facility against her will for an indefinite period of time. The commitment is based on the client's need for psychiatric treatment, the risk of harm to self or others, or the inability to provide self-care. The need for commitment could be determined by a judge of the court or by another agency. The number of physicians required to certify that the client's condition requires commitment varies from state to state (usually two).

  o Emergency involuntary commitment – A type of involuntary commitment in which the client is hospitalized to prevent harm to self or others. Emergency commitment is usually temporary (can be up to 10 days). This type of commitment is usually imposed by providers, mental health providers, or police officers.

    ○   Observational or temporary involuntary commitment – A type of involuntary commitment in which the client is in need of observation, a diagnosis, and a treatment plan. The time for this type of commitment is controlled by state statute and varies greatly among states. This may be imposed by a family member, legal guardian, provider, or a mental health provider.

    ○   Long-term or formal involuntary commitment – A type of commitment that is similar to temporary commitment, but must be imposed by the courts. Time of commitment varies, but is usually 60 to 180 days. Sometimes, there is no set release date.

    ○   Clients admitted under involuntary commitment are still considered competent and have the right to refuse treatment, unless they have gone through a legal competency hearing and have been judged incompetent. The client who has been judged incompetent has a temporary or permanent guardian, usually a family member if possible, appointed by the court. The guardian can sign informed consent for the client. The guardian is expected to consider what the client would want if he were still competent.

Ⓢ Client Rights Regarding Seclusion and Restraint

 View Media Supplement: Restraint Use (Video)

- Nurses must know and follow federal, state, and facility policies that govern the use of restraints.

- Use of seclusion rooms and/or restraints may be warranted and authorized for clients in some cases.

- In general, seclusion and/or restraint should be prescribed for the shortest duration necessary, and only if less restrictive measures are not sufficient. They are for the physical protection of the client and/or other clients and staff.

- A client may voluntarily request temporary seclusion in cases where the environment is disturbing or seems too stimulating.

- Restraints can be either physical (mitt restraint) or chemical (neuroleptic medication) to calm the client.

- Never use seclusion and/or restraint for:

    ○   Convenience of the staff

    ○   Punishment of the client

    ○   Clients who are extremely physically or mentally unstable

    ○   Clients who cannot tolerate the decreased stimulation of a seclusion room

- When all other less restrictive means have been tried to prevent a client from harming self or others, the following must occur in order for seclusion or restraint to be used:

    ○   The treatment must be prescribed by the provider in writing.

    ○   The prescription must specify the duration of treatment.

- ○ The provider must rewrite the prescription, specifying the type of restraint, every 24 hr or as frequently as specified by facility policy.

- ○ Nursing responsibilities must be identified in the protocol, including how often the client should be:

  - ▪ Checked (including for safety and physical needs), and the client's behavior documented

  - ▪ Offered food and fluid

  - ▪ Toileted

  - ▪ Monitored for vital signs

- ○ Complete documentation includes a description of the following:

  - ▪ Precipitating events and behavior of the client prior to seclusion or restraint

  - ▪ Alternative actions taken to avoid seclusion or restraint

  - ▪ The time treatment began

  - ▪ The client's current behavior, what foods or fluids were offered and taken, needs provided for, and vital signs

  - ▪ Medication administration

- • An emergency situation must be present for the charge nurse to use seclusion or restraints without first obtaining a provider's written prescription. If this treatment is initiated, the nurse must obtain the written prescription within a specified period of time (usually 15 to 30 min).

Tort Law in the Mental Health Setting

- • Although intentional torts can occur in any health care setting, they are particularly likely to occur in mental health settings because of the increased likelihood of violence and client behavior that can be challenging to facility staff. Following are examples of torts:

INTENTIONAL TORT	EXAMPLE
False imprisonment	Confining a client to a specific area (a seclusion room) is false imprisonment if the reason for such confinement is for the convenience of the staff.
Assault	Making a threat to a client's person (approaching the client in a threatening manner with a syringe in hand) is considered assault.
Battery	Touching a client in a harmful or offensive way is considered battery. This would occur if the nurse threatening the client with a syringe actually grabbed the client and gave the injection.

Documentation

- It is vital to clearly and objectively document information related to violent or other unusual episodes. The nurse should document:

  - Client behavior in a clear and objective manner.

    - Example: The client suddenly began to run down the hall with both hands in the air, screaming obscenities.

  - Staff response to disruptive, violent, or potentially harmful behavior, such as suicide threats or potential or actual harm to others, including timelines and the extent of response.

    - Example: The client states, "I'm going to pound (other client) into the ground." Client picks up a chair and stands 3 ft from other client with chair held over his head in both hands. Nurse calls for help. Client is immediately told by nurse, "Put down the chair and back away from (the other person)." The other client is moved away to a safe area. Five other staff members respond to the verbal call for help within 30 sec and stand several yards from the client. The client then puts the chair down, quietly turns around, walks to his room, and sits on the bed.

(A) APPLICATION EXERCISES

1. An example of a client who requires emergency admission to a mental health facility is one who has been diagnosed with

    A. paranoid schizophrenia and reports frequent auditory hallucinations.

    B. major depression and attempted suicide 1 year ago.

    C. post-traumatic stress disorder and assaulted his son with a bat.

    D. bipolar disease and paces quickly along the sidewalk.

2. A client tells a nurse, "Don't tell anyone, but I hid a big pair of scissors under my mattress to protect myself from that night janitor, who is always telling me he wants to have sex with me." Which of the following actions should the nurse take?

    A. Keep the client's communication confidential, but talk to the client daily about hiding the scissors.

    B. Keep the client's communication confidential, but watch the client's behavior closely.

    C. Tell the client that this must be reported to the staff because it concerns safety.

    D. Report the incident, but do not inform the client of having the intention to do so.

3. A nurse who decides to place a client who has psychosis in seclusion overnight because the unit is short-staffed and the client is a risk for injury to other clients is displaying behavior representative of

    A. beneficence.

    B. a tort.

    C. a facility policy.

    D. justice.

4. A nurse is caring for a client who is in restraints. Which of the following is appropriate documentation? (Select all that apply.)

    _____ "Client ate very little of his evening snack"

    _____ "Client escorted to the toilet every 2 hr by assistive personnel"

    _____ "Client stated he will "get out of these things and run out the door"

    _____ "Client received haloperidol (Haldol) 2 mg PO at 1800"

    _____ "Client became anxious after dinner"

APPLICATION EXERCISES ANSWER KEY

1. An example of a client who requires emergency admission to a mental health facility is one who has been diagnosed with

    A. paranoid schizophrenia and reports frequent auditory hallucinations.

    B. major depression and attempted suicide 1 year ago.

    C. post-traumatic stress disorder and assaulted his son with a bat.

    D. bipolar disease and paces quickly along the sidewalk.

    The client who has post-traumatic stress disorder and assaulted his son with a bat is a current danger to self or others, and therefore, requires emergency admission to a mental health facility. The presence of auditory hallucinations, symptoms of depression without a recent suicide attempt or intent to commit suicide, and hypermotor activity symptoms are not clear reasons for emergency commitment.

    (N) NCLEX® Connection: Psychosocial Integrity, Crisis Intervention

2. A client tells a nurse, "Don't tell anyone, but I hid a big pair of scissors under my mattress to protect myself from that night janitor, who is always telling me he wants to have sex with me." Which of the following actions should the nurse take?

    A. Keep the client's communication confidential, but talk to the client daily about hiding the scissors.

    B. Keep the client's communication confidential, but watch the client's behavior closely.

    C. Tell the client that this must be reported to the staff because it concerns safety.

    D. Report the incident, but do not inform the client of having the intention to do so.

    This is a serious safety issue, and possibly harassment, that must be reported to the staff. Using the principle of veracity, the nurse should tell this client truthfully what must be done regarding the issue.

    (N) NCLEX® Connection: Safety and Infection Control, Accident/Error/Injury Prevention

3. A nurse who decides to place a client who has psychosis in seclusion overnight because the unit is short-staffed and the client is a risk for injury to other clients is displaying behavior representative of

    A. beneficence.

    B. a tort.

    C. a facility policy.

    D. justice.

    A civil wrong that violates a client's civil rights is a tort, in this case, false imprisonment. The decision is neither beneficence (doing good for a client) nor justice (fair and equal treatment). If this were indeed a facility policy, it would violate a federal and state statute, and the nurse could still be held responsible for following it.

(N) NCLEX® Connection: Safety and Infection Control, Restraints/Safety Devices

4. A nurse is caring for a client who is in restraints. Which of the following is appropriate documentation? (Select all that apply.)

    _____ "Client ate very little of his evening snack"

    __X__ **"Client escorted to the toilet every 2 hr by assistive personnel"**

    __X__ **"Client stated he will "get out of these things and run out the door"**

    __X__ **"Client received haloperidol (Haldol) 2 mg PO at 1800"**

    _____ "Client became anxious after dinner"

How the client's elimination needs were met, the example of the client's verbal communication, and the dosage and time of medication administration are all objective data the nurse should document when caring for a client who is in restraints. The nurse should document exactly how much the client ate and what behaviors the client demonstrated.

(N) NCLEX® Connection: Safety and Infection Control, Restraints/Safety Devices

UNIT 1	FOUNDATIONS FOR MENTAL HEALTH NURSING
Chapter 3	Effective Communication

Overview

- Communication is a complex process of sending, receiving, and comprehending messages between two or more people. It is a dynamic and ongoing process that creates a unique experience between the participants.

  o Communicating effectively is a skill that can be developed.

  o Nurses use communication when providing care to establish relationships, demonstrate caring, obtain information, and assist with changing behaviors.

  o Foundational to the nurse-client relationship is therapeutic communication.

Basic Communication

- Four Primary Levels of Basic Communication

  o Intrapersonal communication – Communication that occurs within an individual. Also identified as "self-talk." This occurs within one's self and is the internal discussion that takes place when an individual is thinking thoughts and not outwardly verbalizing them. In nursing, intrapersonal communication allows the nurse to evaluate a client and/or situation and critically think about the client/situation before communicating verbally.

  o Interpersonal communication – Communication that occurs between two or more people in a small group. This form of communication is the most common in nursing and requires an exchange of information with an individual or small group.

  o Public communication – Communication that occurs within large groups of people. In nursing, this commonly occurs during educational endeavors where the nurse is providing information for a large group of individuals, such as in a community setting.

  o Transpersonal communication – Communication that addresses an individual's spiritual needs and provides interventions to meet those needs.

- Verbal Communication

VERBAL COMMUNICATION	
CONTENT OF THE MESSAGE	IMPACT ON THE COMMUNICATION
Vocabulary – These are the words that are used to communicate either a written or a spoken message.	Limited vocabulary or speaking a language other than English can make it difficult for the nurse to communicate with the client. Use of medical jargon can decrease client understanding.
Denotative/connotative meaning – When communicating, participants must share meanings.	Words that have multiple meanings can cause miscommunication if they are interpreted differently.
Clarity/brevity – The shortest, simplest communication is usually most effective.	Communication that is long and complex can be difficult to understand.
Timing/relevance – Knowing when to communicate allows the receiver to be more attentive to the message.	Communicating with a client who is in pain or distracted will make it difficult for the message to be conveyed.
Pacing – The rate of speech can communicate a meaning to the receiver.	Speaking rapidly may communicate the impression that the nurse is in a rush and does not have time for the client.
Intonation – The tone of voice can communicate a variety of feelings.	The nurse can communicate feelings (acceptance, judgment, dislike) through tone of voice.

- Nonverbal Communication
  - Nurses should be aware of how they communicate nonverbally. The nurse should observe the client's nonverbal communications for the meaning being conveyed, remembering that culture affects interpretation. Attention to the following behaviors is important, as it is compared to the verbal message being conveyed:
    - Appearance
    - Posture
    - Gait
    - Facial expressions
    - Eye contact
    - Gestures
    - Sounds
    - Territoriality
    - Personal space
    - Silence
    - Touch

Therapeutic Communication

- Therapeutic communication is the purposeful use of communication to build and maintain helping relationships with clients, families, and significant others.

- The nurse uses interactive, purposeful communication skills to:

  o Elicit and attend to the client's thoughts, feelings, concerns, and needs.

  o Express empathy and genuine concern for the client's and family's issues.

  o Obtain information and give feedback about the client's condition.

  o Intervene to promote functional behavior and effective interpersonal relationships.

  o Evaluate the client's progress toward goals and outcomes.

- Children and older adults frequently require altered techniques to enhance communication.

- Use of the nursing process depends on therapeutic communication between the nurse, the client, the client's family, and the interdisciplinary care team.

- Characteristics of Therapeutic Communication

  o Client centered – not social or reciprocal

  o Purposeful, planned, and goal-directed

- Essential Components of Therapeutic Communication

  o Time – Plan for and allow adequate time to communicate.

  o Attending behaviors or active listening – These are nonverbal means of conveying interest in another.

    ▪ Eye contact typically conveys interest and respect, but varies by situation and culture.

    ▪ Body language and posture may demonstrate level of comfort and ease.

    ▪ Vocal quality enhances rapport and emphasizes particular topics or issues.

    ▪ Verbal tracking provides feedback by restating or summarizing a client's statements.

  o Caring attitude – Show concern and facilitate an emotional connection with the client and the client's family.

  o Honesty – Be open, direct, truthful, and sincere.

  o Trust – Demonstrate reliability without doubt or question.

  o Empathy – Convey an objective awareness and understanding of the feelings, emotions, and behaviors of others, including trying to envision what it must be like to be in the position of the client and the client's family.

  o Nonjudgmental attitude – This is a display of acceptance that will encourage open, honest communication.

View Media Supplement: Therapeutic and Nontherapeutic Communication (Video)

Nursing Process

- Data Collection
  - ○ Evaluate verbal and nonverbal communication needs.
  - ○ Consider the client's developmental level and how communication should be altered during the data collection phase.
    - Children
      - □ Use simple, straightforward language.
      - □ Be aware of own nonverbal messages, as children are sensitive to nonverbal communication.
      - □ Enhance communication by being at the child's eye level.
      - □ Incorporate play in interactions.
    - Older adult clients
      - □ Recognize that the client may require amplification.
      - □ Minimize distractions, and face the client when speaking.
      - □ Allow plenty of time for the client to respond.
      - □ When impaired communication is identified, ask for input from caregivers or family to determine the extent of the deficits and how best to communicate.
    - Identify any cultural considerations that may affect communication.
- Planning
  - ○ Minimize distractions.
  - ○ Provide for privacy.
  - ○ Identify mutually agreed-upon client outcomes.
  - ○ Set priorities according to the client's needs.
  - ○ Plan for adequate time for interventions.
- Implementation
  - ○ Establish a trusting nurse-client relationship. The client feels more at ease during the implementation phase when a helping relationship has been established.
  - ○ Provide empathetic responses and explanations to the client by using observations and providing hope, humor, and information.

Effective Skills and Techniques

EFFECTIVE COMMUNICATION	INFLUENCE ON COMMUNICATION
Silence	Allows time for meaningful reflection
Active listening	Hear, observe, and understand what clients communicate and provide feedback
Open-ended questions	Facilitate spontaneous responses and interactive discussion
Clarifying techniques	Use to determine if the message received was accurate by: • Restating – Use the client's exact words. • Reflecting – Direct the focus back to the client in order for the client to examine his feelings. • Paraphrasing – Restate the client's feelings and thoughts for the client to confirm what has been communicated. • Exploring – Gather more information regarding important topics mentioned by the client.
Offering general leads and broad opening statements	Encourages clients to determine where the communication can start and to continue talking
Showing acceptance and recognition	Acknowledges the nurse's interest and nonjudgmental attitude
Focusing	Helps clients concentrate on what is important
Asking questions	Offers a way to seek additional information
Giving information	Provides details that clients may need for decision making
Presenting reality	Helps clients focus on what is actually happening and to dispel delusions, hallucinations, or faulty beliefs
Summarizing	Emphasizes important points and reviews what has been discussed
Offering self	Demonstrates a willingness to spend time with clients. Share limited personal information, but return the focus to the client as soon as possible. Relevant self-disclosure by nurses allows clients to see that their experience is shared by others and understood.
Touch	If appropriate, communicates caring and may provide comfort to the client

Barriers to Effective Communication

- Asking irrelevant personal questions
- Offering personal opinions
- Giving advice
- Giving false reassurance
- Minimizing feelings
- Changing the topic

- Asking "why" questions

- Offering value judgments

- Excessive questioning

- Responding approvingly or disapprovingly

- Failure to listen attentively

- Giving conflicting verbal and nonverbal messages

Client Outcomes

- The client will verbalize concerns to the nurse.

- The client will request assistance from the nurse as appropriate.

- The client will communicate needs to the nurse.

APPLICATION EXERCISES

1. Give two examples of how a nurse can use intrapersonal communication to enhance communication with a client.

2. Match the element of verbal communication with the appropriate example that could result in miscommunication.

_____	Pacing	A.	Use of medical jargon the client is unlikely to understand, such as "your labs say to up your meds"
_____	Connotative meaning	B.	Charting that is written "client complains of" vs "client reports"
_____	Vocabulary	C.	A client not asking the nurse a question because the nurse is speaking rapidly and seems very busy
_____	Brevity	D.	A nurse attempting to reinforce teaching about dietary guidelines while the client is falling asleep
_____	Timing	E.	A nurse spending time explaining to the client the intricacies of the multidepartment electronic input and system before the client can be discharged

3. Which of the following is a barrier to therapeutic communication?

   A. Changing the topic

   B. Summarizing

   C. Presenting reality

   D. Offering general leads

4. When a family asks a nurse for reassurance about a client's condition, which of the following is an appropriate response?

   A. "I have seen many families go through this. It gets easier with time."

   B. "I think you need to spend more time just sitting with him. Just tell him you know he'll get better."

   C. "I really can't say what will happen. Have you asked the doctor about this?"

   D. "I understand your need for reassurance. Let's talk about what concerns you specifically."

APPLICATION EXERCISES ANSWER KEY

1. Give two examples of how a nurse can use intrapersonal communication to enhance communication with a client.

   A nurse enters a client's room and sees that the client is crying. Using the technique of self-talk, the nurse asks herself, "I wonder why this client is so upset? Is he sad? Is he in pain? Does he have a social support system?" The nurse's questions then stem from the intrapersonal communication. The nurse is using intrapersonal communication skills to identify a potential problem, and she intervenes by asking the client pertinent questions to come to a more concrete answer.

   A client's condition is deteriorating, and the nurse must phone the provider. Intrapersonally, the nurse goes through a self-talk discussion about what to say to the provider. This allows the nurse to be proactive and to anticipate the provider's requests and questions. The nurse's intrapersonal communication enhances the interpersonal communication with the provider to meet the needs of the client. The nurse is using self-talk to prepare for a future interpersonal communication encounter.

   NCLEX® Connection: Psychosocial Integrity, Therapeutic Communication

2. Match the element of verbal communication with the appropriate example that could result in miscommunication.

C	Pacing	A. Use of medical jargon the client is unlikely to understand, such as "your labs say to up your meds"
B	Connotative meaning	B. Charting that is written "client complains of" vs "client reports"
A	Vocabulary	C. A client not asking the nurse a question because the nurse is speaking rapidly and seems very busy
E	Brevity	D. A nurse attempting to reinforce teaching about dietary guidelines while the client is falling asleep
D	Timing	E. A nurse spending time explaining to the client the intricacies of the multidepartment electronic input and system before the client can be discharged

   NCLEX® Connection: Psychosocial Integrity, Therapeutic Communication

3. Which of the following is a barrier to therapeutic communication?

   A. Changing the topic

   B. Summarizing

   C. Presenting reality

   D. Offering general leads

   Changing the topic should be avoided because it tends to disregard or dismiss the client's feelings or train of thought. Summarizing, on the other hand, encourages the client to consider the important points of the discussion. Presenting reality is therapeutic because it helps the client focus on what is happening in the present situation. Offering general leads encourages the client to continue talking.

   Ⓝ NCLEX® Connection: Psychosocial Integrity, Therapeutic Communications

4. When a family asks a nurse for reassurance about a client's condition, which of the following is an appropriate response?

   A. "I have seen many families go through this. It gets easier with time."

   B. "I think you need to spend more time just sitting with him. Just tell him you know he'll get better."

   C. "I really can't say what will happen. Have you asked the doctor about this?"

   D. "I understand your need for reassurance. Let's talk about what concerns you specifically."

   The therapeutic response reflects and accepts the family's feelings and allows the members to clarify what they are feeling. Other responses interject the nurse's opinion, offer false reassurance, or refer the family elsewhere. These nontherapeutic responses may cause the family to withhold their thoughts and feelings.

   Ⓝ NCLEX® Connection: Psychosocial Integrity, Therapeutic Communication

| UNIT 1 | FOUNDATIONS FOR MENTAL HEALTH NURSING |
| Chapter 4 | Anxiety and Defense Mechanisms |

Overview

- Stress can result from a change in one's environment that is threatening, causes challenges, or is perceived as damaging to that person's well-being. Stress causes anxiety.

- Dysfunctional behavior may occur when a defense mechanism is used as a response to anxiety.

- Individuals may use defense mechanisms as a way to manage conflict in response to anxiety. Defense mechanisms are reversible and can be adaptive, as well as maladaptive.

  ○ Adaptive use of defense mechanisms helps people to achieve their goals in acceptable ways. Defense mechanisms become maladaptive when they interfere with functioning, relationships, and orientation to reality.

  ○ It is important that the defense mechanism used is appropriate to the situation and that an individual uses a variety of defense mechanisms, rather than having the same reaction to every situation.

Defense Mechanisms

- Healthy defenses include altruism, sublimation, humor, and suppression.

- Intermediate defenses include repression, reaction formation, somatization, displacement, rationalization, and undoing.

- Immature defenses include projection, acting-out behaviors, dissociation, devaluation, idealization, splitting, passive aggression, and denial.

DEFENSE MECHANISM	DESCRIPTION	EXAMPLE
Altruism	Dealing with anxiety by reaching out to others	A nurse who lost a family member in a fire is a volunteer firefighter.
Sublimation	Dealing with unacceptable feelings or impulses by unconsciously substituting acceptable forms of expression	A person who has feelings of anger and hostility toward his work supervisor sublimates those feelings by working out vigorously at the gym during his lunch period.
Suppression	Voluntarily denying unpleasant thoughts and feelings	A person who has lost his job states he will worry about paying his bills next week.
Repression	Putting unacceptable ideas, thoughts, and emotions out of conscious awareness	A person who has a fear of the dentist's drill continually "forgets" his dental appointments.

DEFENSE MECHANISM	DESCRIPTION	EXAMPLE
Displacement	Shifting feelings related to an object, person, or situation to another less threatening object, person, or situation	A person who is angry about losing his job destroys his child's favorite toy.
Reaction formation	Overcompensating or demonstrating the opposite behavior of what is felt	A person who dislikes her sister's daughter offers to babysit so that her sister can go out of town.
Somatization	Developing a physical symptom in place of anxiety	A school-age child develops abdominal pain to avoid going to school where he is being bullied.
Undoing	Performing an act to make up for prior behavior	An adolescent completes his chores without being prompted after having an argument with his parent.
Rationalization	Creating reasonable and acceptable explanations for unacceptable behavior	A young adult explains he had to drive home from a party after drinking alcohol because he had to feed his dog.
Passive aggression	Indirectly behaving aggressively, but appearing to be compliant	A person's coworker agrees to take on one of her assignments, but then does not meet the deadline.
Acting-out behaviors	Managing emotional conflicts through actions, rather than self-reflection	A preschool child is told to share her toys, so she throws the toys across the room.
Dissociation	Temporarily blocking memories and perceptions from consciousness	An adolescent witnesses a shooting and is unable to recall any details of the event.
Devaluation	Expressing negative thoughts of self or others	A person who is passed up for a promotion states that the job is not better than the one he currently has.
Idealization	Expressing extremely positive thoughts of self or others	A school-age boy boasts about his older brother and his accomplishments.
Splitting	Demonstrating an inability to reconcile negative and positive attributes of self or others	A client tells a nurse that she is the only one who cares about her, yet the following day, the same client refuses to talk to the nurse.
Projection	Blaming others for unacceptable thoughts and feelings	A young adult blames his substance abuse on his parents' refusal to buy him a new car.
Denial	Pretending the truth is not reality to manage the anxiety of acknowledging what is real	A parent who is informed that his son was killed in combat tells everyone he is coming home for the holidays.

Anxiety

- Anxiety is viewed on a continuum with increasing levels of anxiety leading to decreasing ability to function.

    ○ Normal – A healthy life force that is necessary for survival, normal anxiety motivates people to take action. For example, a potentially violent situation occurs on the mental health unit and the nurse moves rapidly to defuse the situation. The anxiety experienced by the nurse during the situation helped him perform quickly and efficiently.

    ○ Acute (state) – This level of anxiety is precipitated by an imminent loss or change that threatens one's sense of security. For example, the sudden death of a loved one precipitates an acute state of anxiety.

    ○ Chronic (trait) – This level of anxiety is one that usually develops over time, often starting in childhood. The adult who experiences chronic anxiety may display that anxiety in physical symptoms, such as fatigue and frequent headaches.

- Determining a client's level of anxiety is basic to therapeutic intervention in any setting.

LEVELS OF ANXIETY	
Mild	<ul><li>Mild anxiety occurs in the normal experience of everyday living.</li><li>It increases one's ability to perceive reality.</li><li>There is an identifiable cause of the anxiety.</li><li>Other characteristics include a vague feeling of mild discomfort, impatience, and apprehension.</li></ul>
Moderate	<ul><li>Moderate anxiety occurs when mild anxiety escalates.</li><li>Slightly reduced perception and processing of information occurs, and selective inattention may occur.</li><li>Ability to think clearly is hampered, but learning and problem solving may still occur.</li><li>Other characteristics include concentration difficulties, tiredness, pacing, and increased heart rate and respiratory rate.</li><li>Clients with this type of anxiety usually benefits from the direction of others.</li></ul>
Severe	<ul><li>Perceptual field is greatly reduced with distorted perceptions.</li><li>Learning and problem solving do not occur.</li><li>Other characteristics include confusion, feelings of impending doom, and aimless activity.</li><li>Clients with severe anxiety usually are not able to take direction from others.</li></ul>
Panic-level	<ul><li>Panic-level anxiety is characterized by markedly disturbed behavior.</li><li>Clients are not able to process what is occurring in the environment and may lose touch with reality.</li><li>Clients experience extreme fright and horror.</li><li>Other characteristics may include dysfunction in speech, inability to sleep, delusions, and hallucinations.</li></ul>

- Nursing interventions are implemented according to the level of anxiety that clients are experiencing.

NURSING INTERVENTION	THERAPEUTIC INTENT
Nursing interventions for the client with mild to moderate levels of anxiety	
Use active listening to demonstrate willingness to help, and use specific communication techniques (open-ended questions, giving broad openings, exploring, and seeking clarification).	These interventions encourage the client to express feelings, develop trust, and identify the source of the anxiety.
Provide a calm presence, recognizing the client's distress.	This assists the client to focus and to begin problem solving.
Evaluate past coping mechanisms.	This will assist the client to identify adaptive and nonadaptive coping mechanisms.
Explore alternatives to problem situations.	This intervention offers options for problem solving.
Encourage participation in activities, such as exercise, that may temporarily relieve feelings of inner tension.	This provides the client with an outlet for pent-up tension, promotes endorphin release, and improves mental well-being.
Nursing interventions for the client with severe to panic levels of anxiety	
Provide an environment that meets the physical and safety needs of the client. Remain with the client.	This intervention minimizes risk to the client. The client may be unaware of the need for basic things, such as fluids, food, and sleep.
Provide a quiet environment with minimal stimulation.	This helps to prevent intensification of the current level of anxiety.
Use medications and restraint only after less restrictive interventions have failed to decrease anxiety to safer levels.	Medications and/or restraint may be necessary to prevent harm to the client and providers.
Encourage gross motor activities, such as walking and other forms of exercise.	This provides the client with an outlet for pent-up tension, promotes endorphin release, and improves mental well-being.
Set limits by using firm, short, and simple statements. Repetition may be necessary.	Limit-setting can minimize risk to the client and providers. Clear, simple communication facilitates understanding.
Direct clients to acknowledge reality and focus on what is present in the environment.	Focusing on reality will assist in reducing the client's anxiety level.

(A) APPLICATION EXERCISES

1. Match each defense mechanism below with the letter of the behavior that illustrates it.

_____	Suppression	A. A child is punished by his mother and sent to his room, where he begins to kick and break a favorite toy.
_____	Somatization	B. A woman who just lost her job because she frequently was late for work tells friends that it will be much better for her family if she stays home every day.
_____	Displacement	C. A man who is preparing for a presentation at a conference coughs up blood, but waits until after the conference to make an appointment with his provider.
_____	Rationalization	D. A woman who has a fear of flying, but must travel for her job, develops an intense headache whenever she prepares for a flight.
_____	Sublimation	E. A husband feels angry with his wife, so he goes outside and begins energetically cutting up firewood with an axe.

2. A client in his provider's office just learned that he must have prostate surgery. As the nurse tries to reinforce his preoperative instructions, the client becomes agitated. His voice trembles as he says, "I don't know why you are even talking to me. I have not seen you before, and I can't do any of those things you're telling me to do." The nurse documents the client's anxiety as

   A. mild.

   B. moderate.

   C. severe.

   D. panic.

3. Which of the following is an appropriate nursing strategy when trying to give necessary information to a client who has mild anxiety?

   A. Reassure the client that everything will be okay.

   B. Encourage the client to talk about her feelings of anxiety.

   C. Suggest taking a walk together, while reinforcing the information.

   D. Demonstrate a calm manner, while using simple and clear language.

Scenario: A man enters the emergency department with his son, who has just been injured by a motor vehicle. The father was supposed to be watching the 6 year old while the child's mother was shopping; however, the child left the house unnoticed and wandered into the street in front of his home. At the hospital, the child is immediately sent to surgery and is in critical condition. The father, who is still in the emergency department's waiting room, is very distraught and is wailing loudly. He demonstrates an inability to be still, his hands are shaking, and he is frequently dropping his keys. "It should have been me," he moans. Others in the waiting room are starting to appear anxious and are reporting the disturbance.

4. What level of anxiety is the father experiencing? Which data support this description?

5. Identify three nursing interventions for this family member.

(A) APPLICATION EXERCISES ANSWER KEY

1. Match each defense mechanism below with the letter of the behavior that illustrates it.

    C   Suppression

    D   Somatization

    A   Displacement

    B   Rationalization

    E   Sublimation

    A. A child is punished by his mother and sent to his room, where he begins to kick and break a favorite toy.

    B. A woman who just lost her job because she frequently was late for work tells friends that it will be much better for her family if she stays home every day.

    C. A man who is preparing for a presentation at a conference coughs up blood, but waits until after the conference to make an appointment with his provider.

    D. A woman who has a fear of flying, but must travel for her job, develops an intense headache whenever she prepares for a flight.

    E. A husband feels angry with his wife, so he goes outside and begins energetically cutting up firewood with an axe.

(N) NCLEX® Connection: Psychosocial Integrity, Mental Health Concepts

2. A client in his provider's office just learned that he must have prostate surgery. As the nurse tries to reinforce his preoperative instructions, the client becomes agitated. His voice trembles as he says, "I don't know why you are even talking to me. I have not seen you before, and I can't do any of those things you're telling me to do." The nurse documents the client's anxiety as

    A. mild.

    B. moderate.

    C. severe.

    D. panic.

    Severe anxiety causes restlessness, confusion, decreased perception, and an inability to take direction. With mild anxiety, the person's ability to understand information may actually increase. Moderate anxiety decreases problem solving and may hamper the person's ability to understand information. Vital signs may increase somewhat, and the person is visibly anxious. During a panic attack, the person is completely distracted, unable to function, and may lose touch with reality.

(N) NCLEX® Connection: Psychosocial Integrity, Behavioral Management

3. Which of the following is an appropriate nursing strategy when trying to give necessary information to a client who has mild anxiety?

    A. Reassure the client that everything will be okay.

    B. Encourage the client to talk about her feelings of anxiety.

    C. Suggest taking a walk together, while reinforcing the information.

    D. Demonstrate a calm manner, while using simple and clear language.

    Giving information simply and calmly will help the client grasp essential facts. With mild anxiety, the client's ability to understand directions is not impaired and might even increase, so there is no need to alter the process. Offering false reassurance is a nontherapeutic intervention. Trying to make the client verbalize her feelings might distract her from grasping the information. Encouraging gross motor activities is a strategy recommended for clients who have severe or panic levels of anxiety.

 NCLEX® Connection: Psychosocial Integrity, Behavioral Management

Scenario: A man enters the emergency department with his son, who has just been injured by a motor vehicle. The father was supposed to be watching the 6 year old while the child's mother was shopping; however, the child left the house unnoticed and wandered into the street in front of his home. At the hospital, the child is immediately sent to surgery and is in critical condition. The father, who is still in the emergency department's waiting room, is very distraught and is wailing loudly. He demonstrates an inability to be still, his hands are shaking, and he is frequently dropping his keys. "It should have been me," he moans. Others in the waiting room are starting to appear anxious and are reporting the disturbance.

4. What level of anxiety is the father experiencing? Which data support this description?

    This man demonstrates severe anxiety. He has an extremely reduced attention span, he displays psychomotor agitation, and he is yelling.

 NCLEX® Connection: Psychosocial Integrity, Crisis Intervention

5. Identify three nursing interventions for this family member.

    Appropriate interventions include having a staff member stay with the man; providing a safe and secure environment; observing for and responding to themes noted in his communication; assuring him that he is understood; using firm, short, simple statements to communicate with him; escorting him to a quieter, less populated lounge or waiting area; repeating key information as needed; updating him regularly about his son's progress; and addressing comfort and safety needs by providing fluids and opportunities for nutrition.

 NCLEX® Connection: Psychosocial Integrity, Crisis Intervention

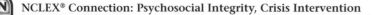

UNIT 1	FOUNDATIONS FOR MENTAL HEALTH NURSING
Chapter 5	Creating and Maintaining a Therapeutic and Safe Environment

Overview

- Therapeutic encounters can occur in any nursing setting if a nurse is sensitive to a client's needs and uses effective communication skills.

- A therapeutic nurse-client relationship is foundational to mental health nursing care.

- A therapeutic nurse-client relationship differs from social and intimate relationships. A therapeutic nurse-client relationship is:

  o Purposeful and goal-directed.

  o Well-defined with clear boundaries.

  o Structured to meet the client's needs.

  o Characterized by an interpersonal process that is safe, confidential, reliable, and consistent.

- Milieu therapy creates an environment that is supportive, therapeutic, and safe.

  o Milieu therapy began as an effort to provide an environment conducive to the treatment of children who were mentally ill.

  o Management of the milieu refers to the management of the total environment of the mental health unit in order to provide the least amount of stress, while promoting the greatest benefit for all the clients.

  o The goal is that while the client is in this therapeutic environment, he will learn the tools necessary to cope adaptively, interact more effectively and appropriately, and strengthen relationship skills. The hope is that the client will use these tools in all other aspects of his life.

  o One structure of the therapeutic milieu is regular community meetings, which include both the clients and the nursing staff.

The Therapeutic Nurse-Client Relationship

- Roles of the Nurse

  o Consistently focus on the client's ideas, experiences, and feelings.

  o Identify and explore the client's needs and problems.

  o Discuss problem-solving alternatives with the client.

  o Help to develop the client's strengths and new coping skills.

  o Encourage positive behavior change in the client.

  o Assist the client to develop a sense of autonomy and self-reliance.

  o Portray genuineness, empathy, and a positive regard toward the client.

- Benefits of a Therapeutic Relationship

  o Therapeutic relationships contribute to the well-being of those who are seriously mentally ill, as well as other clients, although treatment goals are individualized.

  o These relationships take time to establish, but even time-limited therapeutic encounters can have positive outcomes.

  o Therapeutic relationships have a positive impact on the success of treatment.

- Supervision by peers or the clinical team enhances the nurse's ability to examine her own thoughts and feelings, maintain boundaries, and continue to learn from nurse-client relationships.

FACTORS THAT POSITIVELY AFFECT THE DEVELOPMENT OF A THERAPEUTIC RELATIONSHIP	
NURSE FACTORS	CLIENT FACTORS
• Consistent approach to interaction • Adjustment of pace to client's needs • Attentive listening • Positive initial impressions • Comfort level during the relationship • Self-awareness of own thoughts and feelings • Consistent availability	• Trusting attitude • Willingness to talk • Active participation • Consistent availability

PHASES AND TASKS OF A THERAPEUTIC RELATIONSHIP	
NURSE	CLIENT
Orientation Phase	
• Introduce self to the client and state purpose. • Set the contract – Meeting time, place, frequency, duration, and date of termination. • Discuss confidentiality. • Build trust by establishing expectations and boundaries. • Set goals with the client. • Explore the client's ideas, issues, and needs. • Explore the meaning of testing behaviors. • Enforce limits on testing or other inappropriate behaviors.	• Meet with the nurse. • Agree to the contract. • Understand the limits of confidentiality. • Understand the expectations and limits of the relationship. • Participate in setting goals. • Begin to explore own thoughts, experiences, and feelings. • Explore the meaning of own behaviors.
Working Phase	
• Maintain relationship according to the contract. • Perform ongoing data collection to contribute to plan of care and to evaluate therapeutic measures. • Facilitate the client's expression of needs and issues. • Encourage the client to problem solve. • Promote the client's self-esteem. • Foster positive behavioral change. • Explore and deal with resistance and other defense mechanisms. • Recognize transference and countertransference issues. • Reassess the client's problems and goals, and make recommendations for revisions to the plan of care as necessary. • Support the client's adaptive alternatives and use of new coping skills. • Remind the client about the date of termination.	• Explore problematic areas of life. • Reconsider usual coping behaviors. • Examine own worldview and self-concept. • Describe major conflicts and various defenses. • Experience intense feelings, and learn to cope with anxiety reactions. • Test new behaviors. • Begin to develop awareness of transference situations. • Try alternative solutions.

PHASES AND TASKS OF A THERAPEUTIC RELATIONSHIP	
NURSE	CLIENT
Termination Phase	
• Provide opportunity for the client to discuss thoughts and feelings about termination and loss. • Discuss the client's previous experience with separations and loss. • Elicit the client's feelings about the therapeutic work in the nurse-client relationship. • Summarize goals and achievements. • Review memories of work in the sessions. • Express own feelings about sessions to validate the experience with the client. • Discuss ways for the client to incorporate new healthy behaviors into life. • Maintain limits of final termination.	• Discuss thoughts and feelings about termination. • Examine previous separation and loss experiences. • Explore the meaning of the therapeutic relationship. • Review goals and achievements. • Discuss plans to continue new behaviors. • Express any feelings of loss related to termination. • Make plans for the future. • Accept termination as final.

- Boundaries of a Therapeutic Relationship

    o Establish boundaries to maintain a safe and professional nurse-client relationship.

    o Blurred boundaries occur if the relationship begins to meet the needs of the nurse rather than those of the client, or if the relationship becomes social rather than therapeutic.

    o Nurses must work to maintain a consistent level of involvement with clients, to reflect on boundary issues frequently, and to maintain awareness of how behaviors can be perceived by others (clients, family members, other health team members).

TRANSFERENCE AND COUNTERTRANSFERENCE		
DESCRIPTION	EXAMPLE	NURSING IMPLICATIONS
Transference		
Transference occurs when the client views a member of the health care team as having characteristics of another person who has been significant to the client's personal life.	A client may see a nurse as being like his mother, and thus may demonstrate some of the same behaviors with the nurse as he demonstrated with his mother.	Nurses should be aware that transference by clients is more likely to occur with a person in authority.
Countertransference		
Countertransference occurs when a health care team member displaces characteristics of people in her past onto a client.	A nurse may feel defensive and angry with a client for no apparent reason if the client reminds her of a friend who often elicited those feelings.	Nurses should be aware that clients who induce very strong personal feelings may become objects of countertransference.

CHARACTERISTICS OF A THERAPEUTIC MILIEU	
Physical Setting	• A clean and orderly unit • Appropriate color scheme and overall for the client's age • Comfortable furniture placed to promote interaction; solitary spaces for reading and thinking alone; comfortable places conducive to meals; and quiet areas for sleeping • Floors and similar features that are attractive, easy to clean, and safe • Traffic-flow conducive to client and staff movement
Health Care Team Member Responsibilities	• Promote independence for self-care and individual growth in clients. • Treat clients as individuals. • Allow choices for clients within the daily routine and within individual treatment plans. • Apply rules of fair treatment for all clients. • Model good social behavior for clients, such as respect for the rights of others. • Work cooperatively as a team to provide care. • Maintain boundaries with clients. • Maintain a professional appearance and demeanor. • Promote safe and satisfying peer interactions among the clients. • Practice open communication techniques with health team members and clients. • Promote feelings of self-worth and hope for the future.
Emotional climate	• Clients should feel safe from harm (self-harm, harm from disruptive behaviors of other clients). • Clients should feel cared for and accepted by the staff and others.

- Physical Safety

  o The nurses' station and other areas should be placed to allow for easy observation of clients by staff and access to staff by clients.

  o Special safety features, such as bathroom bars and wheelchair accessibility for clients who are disabled, should be addressed.

  o Set up the following provisions to prevent client self-harm or harm by others:

    ▪ No access to sharp or otherwise harmful objects

    ▪ Restriction of client access to restricted or locked areas

    ▪ Monitoring of visitors

    ▪ Restriction of alcohol and illegal drug access or use

    ▪ Restriction of sexual activity among clients

    ▪ Deterrence of elopement from facility

    ▪ Rapid de-escalation of disruptive and potentially violent behaviors through planned interventions by trained staff

○ Seclusion rooms and restraints should be set up for safety and used only after all less restrictive measures have been exhausted. When used, facility policies and procedures must be followed.

○ Plan for safe access to recreational areas, occupational therapy, and meeting rooms.

○ Reinforce fire, evacuation, and other safety rules to all staff.

  ■ Have clear plans for keeping clients and staff safe in emergencies.

  ■ Maintain staff skills, such as cardiopulmonary resuscitation.

○ Considerations of room assignments on a 24-hr inpatient unit should include:

  ■ Personalities of each roommate

  ■ The likelihood of nighttime disruptions for a roommate if one client has difficulty sleeping

  ■ Medical diagnoses, such as how two clients with severe paranoia might interact with each other

○ Activities within the therapeutic milieu are structured and include time for the following:

  ■ Community meetings

    □ The community meeting on the mental health unit should enhance the emotional climate of the therapeutic milieu by promoting:

      ‣ Interaction and communication between staff and clients

      ‣ Decision-making skills of clients

      ‣ A feeling of self-worth among clients

      ‣ Discussions of common unit objectives, such as encouraging clients to meet treatment goals and plan for discharge

      ‣ Discussion of issues of concern to all members of the unit, including common problems, future activities, and the introduction of new clients to the unit

    □ Meetings may be structured so that they are client-led with decisions made by the group as a whole.

  ■ Individual therapy – Scheduled sessions with a mental health provider to address specific mental health concerns, such as depression

  ■ Group therapy – Scheduled sessions for a group of clients to address common mental health issues, such as substance abuse

  ■ Psychoeducational groups – Based on a client's level of functioning and personal needs, such as medication side effects

  ■ Recreational activities, such as a game or a community outing

  ■ Unstructured, flexible time that includes opportunities for the nurse and other staff to observe clients as they interact spontaneously within the milieu

Ⓐ APPLICATION EXERCISES

1. A client says to the nurse, "Why should I talk to you? Everybody knows talking doesn't help!" Which of the following is an appropriate response by the nurse?

   A. "Did someone on the unit tell you that?"

   B. "I'll help if you talk about what's important."

   C. "Why do you think that talking won't help?"

   D. "I'm here to talk with you about your concerns."

2. A nurse is caring for a client who follows her around the unit and tries to engage her in conversation, despite the nurse setting up a specific time for interaction. The client's behavior is an example of which of the following?

   A. Regression to an earlier time

   B. Boredom

   C. Inability to accept limits

   D. Loneliness

3. Which of the following are characteristics of a nurse-client relationship? (Select all that apply.)

   _____ It addresses socialization of both participants.

   _____ It is structured to meet the client's needs.

   _____ Its boundaries are flexible and dynamic.

   _____ It is purposeful and goal-directed.

   _____ It employs a consistent interpersonal process.

4. The working phase of a nurse-client relationship focuses on which of the following?

   A. Encouraging the client to problem solve

   B. Identifying the client's feelings about the therapeutic work

   C. Developing mutually agreeable goals

   D. Exploring the meaning of testing behaviors

5. A nurse is orienting a newly admitted client to an inpatient mental health unit. When explaining the unit's community meetings, the nurse should state which of the following to the client?

   A. "You and a group of other clients will meet to discuss your medication and treatment plans."

   B. "I rarely know what goes on at a community meeting, because the clients control the agenda."

   C. "You and the other clients will meet with staff to discuss activities, problems, and other things of interest to all."

   D. "You and your therapist will meet to discuss your treatment plan and the problems you are having."

APPLICATION EXERCISES ANSWER KEY

1. A client says to the nurse, "Why should I talk to you? Everybody knows talking doesn't help!" Which of the following is an appropriate response by the nurse?

    A. "Did someone on the unit tell you that?"

    B. "I'll help if you talk about what's important."

    C. "Why do you think that talking won't help?"

    D. "I'm here to talk with you about your concerns."

    The correct answer is a broad opening that focuses on the client's feelings and needs. Option A distracts the client from the therapeutic intent of talking. Option B implies that the client is somehow at fault when communicating. Option C implies criticism of the client's response, which could possibly make the client defensive.

 NCLEX® Connection: Psychosocial Integrity, Therapeutic Communication

2. A nurse is caring for a client who follows her around the unit and tries to engage her in conversation, despite the nurse setting up a specific time for interaction. The client's behavior is an example of which of the following?

    A. Regression to an earlier time

    B. Boredom

    C. Inability to accept limits

    D. Loneliness

    Limits must be set so that one client will not monopolize the nurse's time. This may be a boundary issue for the client and nurse. There is no evidence that this is a sign of regression, boredom, or loneliness.

 NCLEX® Connection: Psychosocial Integrity, Therapeutic Environment

3. Which of the following are characteristics of a nurse-client relationship? (Select all that apply.)

    _____ It addresses socialization of both participants.

    __X__ **It is structured to meet the client's needs.**

    _____ Its boundaries are flexible and dynamic.

    __X__ **It is purposeful and goal-directed.**

    __X__ **It employs a consistent interpersonal process.**

    For a nurse-client relationship to be therapeutic and beneficial for the client, it must be focused on the client's needs; purposeful and directed toward goals the nurse and client work toward; and consistent in process. Socialization is the purpose of a social, not a therapeutic, relationship. In a therapeutic relationship, the boundaries must be clear and well-defined.

 NCLEX® Connection: Psychosocial Integrity, Therapeutic Environment

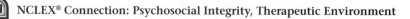

4. The working phase of a nurse-client relationship focuses on which of the following?

   A. Encouraging the client to problem solve

   B. Identifying the client's feelings about the therapeutic work

   C. Developing mutually agreeable goals

   D. Exploring the meaning of testing behaviors

   The working phase is the period of time when the nurse and the client explore behavioral problems, devise and practice new problem-solving skills, and promote positive change. The termination phase is the appropriate time for identifying the client's feelings about the therapeutic work the nurse and client have done together. Developing goals and exploring the meaning of testing behaviors should take place in the orientation phase.

   Ⓝ NCLEX® Connection: Psychosocial Integrity, Therapeutic Environment

5. A nurse is orienting a newly admitted client to an inpatient mental health unit. When explaining the unit's community meetings, the nurse should state which of the following to the client?

   A. "You and a group of other clients will meet to discuss your medication and treatment plans."

   B. "I rarely know what goes on at a community meeting, because the clients control the agenda."

   C. "You and the other clients will meet with staff to discuss activities, problems, and other things of interest to all."

   D. "You and your therapist will meet to discuss your treatment plan and the problems you are having."

   Community meetings include both staff and clients on a unit. Any topic of interest to the entire group may be discussed, including problems, future activities, and meeting newly admitted clients. Option A describes a psychoeducational group. Option B is an evasive answer, as it gives the client no information about meetings. Option D describes individual therapy.

   Ⓝ NCLEX® Connection: Psychosocial Integrity, Therapeutic Environment

UNIT 2: TRADITIONAL NONPHARMACOLOGIC THERAPIES

- Psychoanalysis, Psychotherapy, and Behavioral Therapies
- Group and Family Therapy
- Stress Management
- Electroconvulsive Therapy

NCLEX® CONNECTIONS

When reviewing the chapters in this section, keep in mind the relevant sections of the NCLEX® outline, in particular:

CLIENT NEEDS: HEALTH PROMOTION AND MAINTENANCE	CLIENT NEEDS: PSYCHOSOCIAL INTEGRITY	CLIENT NEEDS: REDUCTION OF RISK POTENTIAL

Relevant topics/tasks include:
- Health Promotion/Disease Prevention
  - Identify risk factors for disease/illness.
- High Risk Behaviors
  - Assist client to identify high risk behaviors.
	Relevant topics/tasks include:
	- Behavioral Management
	  - Participate in client group session.
	- Coping Mechanisms
	  - Identify client support systems and available resources.
	- Stress management
	  - Implement measures to reduce environmental stressors.
		Relevant topics/tasks include:
		- Potential for Complications of Diagnostic Tests/Treatments/Procedures
		  - Provide care for client receiving electroconvulsive therapy.

UNIT 2	TRADITIONAL NONPHARMACOLOGIC THERAPIES
Chapter 6	Psychoanalysis, Psychotherapy, and Behavioral Therapies

Overview

- Psychoanalysis, psychotherapy, and behavioral therapies are approaches to addressing mental health issues using various methods and theoretical bases.

- Nurses working in mental health settings should be familiar with the methods employed among these approaches and how they are applied in practice.

Psychoanalysis

- Classical psychoanalysis is a therapeutic process of assessing unconscious thoughts and feelings, and resolving conflict through talking to a psychoanalyst for many sessions and over months to years.

  o Due to the length of psychoanalytic therapy and health insurance constraints, classical psychoanalysis is less likely to be used as the sole therapy of choice.

  o Psychoanalysis was first developed by Sigmund Freud in order to resolve internal conflicts, which Freud contended always occur from early childhood experiences.

  o Past relationships are a common focus for therapy.

- Therapeutic tools include:

  o Free association, which is the spontaneous, uncensored verbalization of whatever comes to a client's mind

  o Dream analysis and interpretation

  o Transference, which includes feelings that clients have developed toward the therapist related to similar feelings toward significant persons in the client's early childhood

  o Use of defense mechanisms

Psychotherapy

- Psychotherapy involves more verbal therapist-to-client interaction than classic psychoanalysis.

  o A trusting relationship is developed between the client and the therapist in order to explore the client's problems.

  o Psychodynamic psychotherapy employs the same tools as psychoanalysis, but is oriented more to the client's present state, rather than his early life.

- ○ Interpersonal psychotherapy (IPT) is used for clients who have specific problems. It can improve interpersonal relationships, communication, role-relationship, and bereavement.

- ○ Cognitive therapy is based on the cognitive model, which focuses on individual thoughts and behaviors to solve current problems. It is used to treat depression, anxiety, eating disorders, and other issues that can be improved by changing a client's attitude toward life experiences.

- ○ Behavioral therapy

  - ■ In protest of Freud's psychoanalytic theory, behavioral theorists such as Ivan Pavlov, John B. Watson, and B.F. Skinner felt that changing behavior was the key to treating problems such as anxiety and depression.

  - ■ Behavioral therapy is based on the theory that behavior is learned and has consequences. Abnormal behavior results from an attempt to avoid painful feelings. Changing abnormal or maladaptive behavior can occur without the need for insight into the underlying cause of the behavior.

  - ■ Behavioral therapies teach clients ways to decrease anxiety or avoidant behavior and give clients an opportunity to practice techniques.

  - ■ Behavioral therapy has been used successfully to treat clients with phobias, addictions, and other issues.

- ○ Cognitive-behavioral therapy uses both a cognitive and behavioral approach to assist a client with anxiety management.

Use of Cognitive Therapy

- • Cognitive Reframing

  - ○ Anxiety can be decreased by changing cognitive distortions. Cognitive reframing assists clients to identify negative thoughts that produce anxiety, examine the cause, and develop supportive ideas that replace negative self-talk. For example, a client who is depressed may say he is "a bad person" who has "never done anything good" in his life. Through therapy, this client may change his thinking to realize that he may have made some bad choices, but that he is not "a bad person."

    - ■ Priority restructuring – Assists clients to identify what should be given priority, such as devoting energy to pleasurable activities

    - ■ Journal keeping – Helps clients write down stressful thoughts and has a positive effect on well-being

    - ■ Assertiveness training – Teaches clients to express feelings and solve problems in a nonaggressive manner

    - ■ Monitoring thoughts – Helps clients to be aware of negative thinking

Types and Uses of Behavioral Therapy

TYPE	DEFINITION	USE IN MENTAL HEALTH NURSING
Modeling	The therapist or others serve as role models for the client, who learns improved behavior by imitation.	Modeling has been used in the acute care milieu to help clients improve interpersonal skills. The therapist demonstrates appropriate behavior in a stressful situation with the goal of having the client imitate the behavior.
Operant conditioning	Positive rewards are given for positive behavior (positive reinforcement).	Example: Tokens are given to clients for good behavior, and they can be exchanged by the client for a privilege or other items.
Systematic desensitization	This therapy is the planned, progressive, or graduated exposure to anxiety-provoking stimuli in real-life situations or by imagining events that cause anxiety. During this exposure, the anxiety response is suppressed through the use of relaxation techniques.	Systematic desensitization begins with the client mastering relaxation techniques. Then the client is exposed to increasing levels of the anxiety-producing stimulus (either imagined or real) and uses relaxation to overcome anxiety. The client is then able to tolerate a greater and greater level of the stimulus until anxiety no longer interferes with functioning.
Aversion therapy	A maladaptive behavior is paired with a punishment or unpleasant stimuli to change the behavior.	A therapist or treatment team may use unpleasant stimuli (bitter taste, mild electric shock) as punishment for undesired behaviors (alcoholism, violence, self-mutilation, thumb sucking).
Meditation, guided imagery, diaphragmatic breathing, muscle relaxation, and biofeedback	Various techniques are used to control pain, tension, and anxiety.	Example: A nurse can reinforce teaching about diaphragmatic breathing to a client having a panic attack or to a female client in labor.

- Other techniques include:
    - Flooding – Exposing a client, while accompanied by a therapist, to a great deal of an undesirable stimulus in an attempt to turn off the anxiety response
    - Response prevention – Preventing a client from performing a compulsive behavior with the intent that anxiety will be diminished
    - Thought stopping – Telling a client when negative thoughts or compulsive behaviors arise to say or shout, "stop," and substitute a positive thought. The goal over time is for the client to use the command silently.

Ⓐ APPLICATION EXERCISES

1. A client newly admitted to an acute-care locked mental health unit refuses to attend group meetings and will not speak to other clients or attend activities on the unit. She enjoys one-to-one visits with staff and requests to take a walk outside of the building every day with a staff member. During a treatment team meeting, the client's therapist suggests that behavioral therapy might change her negative behavior, and she agrees to try to be more cooperative.

   Explain how behavioral therapy could be used to help the client.

2. A client states that he is depressed because he has had to deal with role reversal with his spouse after the loss of his job due to a disability. Which of the following therapies should the nurse expect to help implement for the client?

   A. Operant conditioning

   B. Systematic desensitization

   C. Psychodynamic psychotherapy

   D. Interpersonal psychotherapy

3. An advanced-practice nurse who uses cognitive reframing is working with a client whose 16-year-old son has run away from home several times in the past year. The client feels that her son's problems are her fault because she is a poor mother. The nurse will use cognitive therapy by

   A. encouraging her to meditate to promote relaxation.

   B. helping her identify and replace negative thoughts.

   C. focusing on her unconscious thoughts related to early childhood.

   D. serving as a positive role model for her.

4. A client in an acute-care mental health facility has depression and will not get out of his bed. Which of the following actions should the nurse take?

   A. Give positive reinforcement for any activity.

   B. Withhold rewards as long as he stays in bed.

   C. Restrict the client's access to his bed.

   D. Insist that the client change his attitude and get up.

5. Match each type of therapy with the example that describes its use.

_____ Psychoanalysis	A. A client who has had heated disputes with other clients on the unit learns to solve problems by sitting down and talking calmly and reasonably with other clients.
_____ Cognitive technique	B. The client discusses his dreams with the therapist.
_____ Assertiveness training	C. The client is encouraged to stop sucking his thumb by having a bitter liquid applied to his thumb.
_____ Aversion therapy	D. A client who feels awkward in group social situations watches a video showing some positive ways to interact in groups.
_____ Modeling	E. A client who displayed violent behavior in the past and felt negative about herself learns to think and speak about herself in more positive terms.

APPLICATION EXERCISES ANSWER KEY

1. A client newly admitted to an acute-care locked mental health unit refuses to attend group meetings and will not speak to other clients or attend activities on the unit. She enjoys one-to-one visits with staff and requests to take a walk outside of the building every day with a staff member. During a treatment team meeting, the client's therapist suggests that behavioral therapy might change her negative behavior, and she agrees to try to be more cooperative.

    Explain how behavioral therapy could be used to help the client.

    The client could use tokens or certificates given as rewards for any positive change of behavior to purchase items she likes. She could use a larger number of tokens or certificates to earn a walk outside with a staff member. Also, giving positive feedback and encouragement for positive behavior may help.

 NCLEX® Connection: Psychosocial Integrity, Behavioral Management

2. A client states that he is depressed because he has had to deal with role reversal with his spouse after the loss of his job due to a disability. Which of the following therapies should the nurse expect to help implement for the client?

    A. Operant conditioning

    B. Systematic desensitization

    C. Psychodynamic psychotherapy

    D. Interpersonal psychotherapy

    Interpersonal psychotherapy will help this client deal with the depression that resulted from the interpersonal problem of role change. Operant conditioning and systematic desensitization are both behavioral therapies that would focus on changing the client's behavior. Psychodynamic psychotherapy would focus on examining unconscious information related to the client's concern.

 NCLEX® Connection: Psychosocial Integrity, Behavioral Management

3. An advanced-practice nurse who uses cognitive reframing is working with a client whose 16-year-old son has run away from home several times in the past year. The client feels that her son's problems are her fault because she is a poor mother. The nurse will use cognitive therapy by

    A. encouraging her to meditate to promote relaxation.

    B. helping her identify and replace negative thoughts.

    C. focusing on her unconscious thoughts related to early childhood.

    D. serving as a positive role model for her.

    Cognitive reframing helps clients replace irrational or unrealistic cognitions (thoughts) with thoughts that are more realistic and positive. Promoting relaxation and acting as a role model are behavioral therapy techniques. Focusing on unconscious thoughts related to early childhood is a technique of psychoanalysis.

 NCLEX® Connection: Psychosocial Integrity, Behavioral Management

4. A client in an acute-care mental health facility has depression and will not get out of his bed. Which of the following actions should the nurse take?

   A. Give positive reinforcement for any activity.

   B. Withhold rewards as long as he stays in bed.

   C. Restrict the client's access to his bed.

   D. Insist that the client change his attitude and get up.

   Giving positive reinforcement is a helpful technique in gradually changing negative behavior. The other options are negative techniques, which are unlikely to encourage any positive behavior.

   Ⓝ NCLEX® Connection: Psychosocial Integrity, Behavioral Management

5. Match each type of therapy with the example that describes its use.

B	Psychoanalysis	A. A client who has had heated disputes with other clients on the unit learns to solve problems by sitting down and talking calmly and reasonably with other clients.
E	Cognitive technique	B. The client discusses his dreams with the therapist.
A	Assertiveness training	C. The client is encouraged to stop sucking his thumb by having a bitter liquid applied to his thumb.
C	Aversion therapy	D. A client who feels awkward in group social situations watches a video showing some positive ways to interact in groups.
D	Modeling	E. A client who displayed violent behavior in the past and felt negative about herself learns to think and speak about herself in more positive terms.

   Ⓝ NCLEX® Connection: Psychosocial Integrity, Behavioral Management

UNIT 2	TRADITIONAL NONPHARMACOLOGIC THERAPIES
Chapter 7	Group and Family Therapy

Overview

- Therapy is an intensive treatment that involves open therapeutic communication with participants who are willing to be involved in therapy.

- Although individual therapy is used as an important treatment for mental illness, group and/or family therapies are also indicated as part of the treatment plan for many clients in a mental health setting.

- Group and family therapy are guided by leaders, who employ leadership styles, such as:

  o Democratic – This style supports group interaction and decision making to solve problems.

  o Laissez-faire – The group process progresses without any attempt by the leader to control the direction of the group.

  o Autocratic – The leader completely controls the direction and structure of the group without allowing group interaction or decision-making to solve problems.

- Examples of group therapy include stress management, chemical/alcohol dependency, medication education, understanding mental illness, and dual diagnosis groups.

Group Therapy

- Group process is the verbal and nonverbal communication that occurs within the group during group sessions.

- Group norm is the way the group behaves during sessions, and over time it provides structure for the group. For example, a group norm could be that members raise their hand to be recognized by the leader before they speak. Another norm could be that all members sit in the same places for each session.

- Hidden agenda – Some group members (or the leader) may have goals different from the stated group goals that may disrupt group processes. For example, three members may try to embarrass another member whom they dislike.

- A subgroup is a small number of people within a larger group who function separately from the group.

- Groups may be open (new members added as old members leave) or closed (no new members added after the group is formed).

- A homogenous group is one in which all members share a certain chosen characteristic, such as diagnosis or gender. Membership of heterogeneous groups is not based on a shared chosen personal characteristic. An example of a heterogeneous group is all clients on a given unit, including a mixture of males and females with a wide range of diagnoses.

- All therapy sessions should include:

    o   The use of open and clear communication

    o   Cohesiveness and guidelines for the therapy session

    o   Direction toward a particular goal

    o   Opportunities for the development of interpersonal skills, resolution of personal and/or family issues, and the development of appropriate, satisfying relationships

    o   Encouragement of the client to maximize positive interactions, feel empowered to make decisions, and strengthen feelings of self-worth

    o   Communication regarding respect among all members

    o   Support, as well as education regarding things such as available community resources for support

- Group therapy goals include:

    o   Sharing of common feelings and concerns

    o   Sharing of stories and experiences

    o   Diminishing feelings of isolation

    o   Creating a community of healing and restoration

    o   Providing a more cost-effective environment than that of individual therapy

- Group therapy may be used for varying age groups.

    o   For children, it is in the form of play while talking about a common experience.

    o   For the adolescent, it is especially valuable, as that age group typically has strong peer relationships.

    o   For the older adult, group therapy helps with socialization and sharing of memories.

PHASES OF GROUP DEVELOPMENT		
PHASE	MAJOR ISSUES	RESPONSIBILITIES
Initial Phase	The purpose and goals of the group are defined.	• The group leader sets a tone of respect, trust, and confidentiality among members. • Members become acquainted with each other and with the group leader. • Termination is discussed.
Working Phase	Problem-solving skills are promoted to facilitate behavioral changes. Power and control issues may dominate in this phase.	• The group leader uses therapeutic communication to encourage group work toward meeting goals. • Members take informal roles within the group, which may interfere with or favor group progress toward goals.
Termination Phase	This marks the end of group sessions.	• Termination issues are discussed among group members. • The leader summarizes work of the group and individual contributions.

- Members of a group can take on a number of roles, including:

  o Maintenance roles – Members who take on these roles tend to help maintain the purpose and process of the group. For example, the harmonizer attempts to prevent conflict in the group.

  o Task roles – Members take on various tasks within the group process. An example of a task role is the recorder, who takes notes and/or records what occurs during each session.

  o Individual roles – These roles tend to prevent teamwork because individuals take on roles to promote their own agenda. Examples include the dominator, who tries to control other members, and the recognition-seeker, who boasts about personal achievements.

Characteristics of Families

- Families may have healthy or dysfunctional characteristics in one or more areas of functioning.

AREA OF FUNCTIONING	HEALTHY FAMILIES	DYSFUNCTIONAL FAMILIES

Communication	There are clear, understandable messages between family members, and each member is encouraged to express individual feelings and thoughts.	• One or more members use unhealthy patterns, such as:
		
		  o Blaming – Members blame others to shift focus away from their own inadequacies.
		
		  o Manipulating – Members use dishonesty to support their own agendas.
		
		  o Placating – One member takes responsibility for problems in order to keep peace at all costs.
		
		  o Distracting – A member inserts irrelevant information during attempts at problem-solving.

Management	Adults of a family agree on important issues, such as rule-making, finances, and plans for the future.	• Management may be chaotic, with a child making management decisions at times.
Boundaries	Boundaries are distinguishable between family roles. Clear boundaries define roles of each member and are understood by all. Each family member is able to function appropriately.	• Enmeshed boundaries – Thoughts, roles, and feelings are so blended that individual roles are unclear. • Rigid boundaries – Rules and roles are completely inflexible. These families tend to have isolated members.
Socialization	All members interact, plan, and adopt healthy ways of coping. Children learn to function as family members, as well as members of society. Members are able to change as the family grows and matures.	• Children do not learn healthy socialization skills within the family and have difficulty adapting to socialization roles of society.
Emotional/ Supportive	Emotional needs of family members are met most of the time, and members are concerned about each other. Conflict and anger do not dominate.	• Negative emotions predominate most of time. Members are isolated and afraid and do not show concern for each other.

- Other concepts related to family dysfunction include:

  o Scapegoating – A member of the family with little power is blamed for problems within the family. For example, one child who has not completed his chores may be blamed for the entire family not being able to go on an outing.

      ○   Triangulation – A third party is drawn into the relationship with two members whose relationship is unstable. For example, one parent may become strongly allied with a child, leaving the other parent relatively uninvolved with both.

      ○   Multigenerational issues – These are emotional issues or themes within a family that continue for at least three generations, such as a pattern of addiction when the family is under stress, dysfunctional grief patterns, triangulation patterns, and divorce.

Family Therapy

- A family is defined as a group with reciprocal relationships in which members are committed to each other. Examples of a family vary widely and are often nontraditional, such as a family made up of a child living with her grown brother and his wife. Areas of functioning for families include management, boundaries, communication, emotional support, and socialization. Dysfunction can occur in any one or more areas.

- In family therapy, the focus is on the family as a system, rather than on each person as an individual.

- Family assessments include focused interviews and use of various family assessment tools.

- Nurses work with families to provide teaching. For example, an RN might instruct a family on medication administration, or ways to provide symptom management for a family member with a mental health disorder.

- Nurses also work to mobilize family resources, improve communication, and strengthen the family's ability to cope with the illness of one member.

FOCUS AND GOALS FOR INDIVIDUAL, FAMILY, AND GROUP THERAPIES		
THERAPY	FOCUS	GOALS
Individual	• Client needs and problems • The therapeutic relationship	• Make more positive individual decisions. • Make productive life decisions. • Develop a strong sense of self.
Family	• Family needs and problems within family dynamics • Improving family functioning	• Learn effective ways for dealing with mental illness within the family. • Improve understanding among family members. • Maximize positive interaction among family members.

Group	• Helping individuals develop more functional and satisfying relations within a group setting	• Goals vary depending on type of group, but clients generally:
		  ○ Discover that members share some common feelings, experiences, and thoughts.
		  ○ Experience positive behavior changes as a result of group interaction and feedback.

Ⓐ APPLICATION EXERCISES

1. A client who has bipolar disorder is active in individual and family therapy. A nurse co-leads the family therapy session. The client expresses concern that his family does not understand his mental illness. The client's family expresses concern that the client may not be responding to the medication. What educational and therapeutic interventions should the nurse perform for the client and the family?

2. A nurse leading a stress management group demonstrates that he supports group interaction and the decision-making required to solve problems. The group proceeds with all members feeling that they have input into the group's decisions. Which leadership style does this illustrate?

    A. Democratic

    B. Laissez-faire

    C. Autocratic

    D. Authoritative

3. A nurse on an acute care mental health unit is helping members learn how to self-manage their psychotropic medications. Several members of the group have decided that they want group members to present information about their own medications. They interrupt the leader repeatedly to tell the other members about their own experiences with medications. This is an example of which of the following?

    A. Homogenous group

    B. Group process

    C. Subgroup

    D. Hidden agenda

4. A nurse is conducting a family therapy session. The teenage son tells the nurse that his parents will punish him harshly if he discloses anything in the session about the family's arguments at home. The parents have never made any such threats to him. This is an example of which of the following?

    A. Placation

    B. Manipulation

    C. Blaming

    D. Distraction

(A) APPLICATION EXERCISES ANSWER KEY

1. A client who has bipolar disorder is active in individual and family therapy. A nurse co-leads the family therapy session. The client expresses concern that his family does not understand his mental illness. The client's family expresses concern that the client may not be responding to the medication. What educational and therapeutic interventions should the nurse perform for the client and the family?

   Try to determine why the family feels the client is not responding to his medications.

   Address the client's and family's concerns and fears.

   Encourage both the client and the family to clarify their concerns.

   Help the client and the family to find strengths on which to build.

   Maintain a nonmanipulative and decentralized communicative environment.

   Provide a safe environment for the client.

   Reinforce teaching that includes medication education.

(N) NCLEX® Connection: Psychosocial Integrity, Support Systems

2. A nurse leading a stress management group demonstrates that he supports group interaction and the decision-making required to solve problems. The group proceeds with all members feeling that they have input into the group's decisions. Which leadership style does this illustrate?

   A. Democratic
   B. Laissez-faire
   C. Autocratic
   D. Authoritative

   A democratic or participative style supports group interaction and decision-making to solve problems. With a laissez-faire style, the group process progresses without any attempt by the leader to control the direction of the group. An autocratic or authoritative leader completely controls the direction and structure of the group without allowing group interaction or decision-making to solve problems.

(N) NCLEX® Connection: Psychosocial Integrity, Behavioral Management

3. A nurse on an acute care mental health unit is helping members learn how to self-manage their psychotropic medications. Several members of the group have decided that they want group members to present information about their own medications. They interrupt the leader repeatedly to tell the other members about their own experiences with medications. This is an example of which of the following?

    A. Homogenous group

    B. Group process

    C. Subgroup

    D. Hidden agenda

    A hidden agenda is what some group members have when their goal differs from that of the group's established goals; this goal is often hidden from some other group members. A homogenous group is one in which all members share a certain chosen characteristic, such as diagnosis or gender. Group process is the verbal and nonverbal communication within the group during group sessions. A subgroup is a small number of people within a larger group who function separately from that group.

    Ⓝ NCLEX® Connection: Psychosocial Integrity, Behavioral Management

4. A nurse is conducting a family therapy session. The teenage son tells the nurse that his parents will punish him harshly if he discloses anything in the session about the family's arguments at home. The parents have never made any such threats to him. This is an example of which of the following?

    A. Placation

    B. Manipulation

    C. Blaming

    D. Distraction

    Manipulation is an attempt to control the situation by dishonest influence rather than through open and honest communication. Placation is a way to maintain harmony in the family. Blaming is done to move the focus to another to prevent being blamed for one's own actions. Distraction is a way to prevent looking at one's own faults by introducing other issues.

    Ⓝ NCLEX® Connection: Psychosocial Integrity, Behavioral Management

| UNIT 2 | TRADITIONAL NONPHARMACOLOGIC THERAPIES |
| Chapter 8 | Stress Management |

Overview

- Stress is the body's nonspecific response to any demand made upon it.

    o Stressors are physical or psychological factors that produce stress. Any stressor, whether it is perceived as "good" or "bad," produces a biological response in the body.

    o Individuals need the presence of some stressors to provide interest and purpose to life; however, too much stress or too many stressors can cause distress.

    o Anxiety and anger are damaging stressors that cause distress.

- General adaptation syndrome (GAS) is the body's response to an increased demand. The first stage is the initial adaptive response, also known as the "fight or flight" mechanism. If stress is prolonged, maladaptive responses can occur.

- Stress management is a person's ability to experience appropriate emotions and cope with stress.

    o The person who manages stress in a healthy manner is flexible and uses a variety of coping techniques or mechanisms.

    o Responses to stress and anxiety are affected by factors such as age, gender, culture, life experiences, and lifestyle.

    o The effects of stressors are cumulative. For example, the death of a family member may cause a high amount of stress. If the person experiencing that stress is also experiencing other stressful events at the same time, this could cause illness due to the cumulative effect of those stressors.

Data Collection

- Protective factors increasing a person's resilience or ability to resist the effects of stress include:

    o Physical health

    o Strong sense of self

    o Religious or spiritual beliefs

    o Optimism

    o Hobbies and other outside interests

- o   Satisfying interpersonal relationships

- o   Strong social support systems

- o   Humor

- Subjective and Objective Data

ACUTE STRESS (FIGHT OR FLIGHT)	PROLONGED STRESS (MALADAPTIVE RESPONSE)
Apprehension	Chronic anxiety or panic attacks
Unhappiness or sorrow	Depression, chronic pain, or sleep disturbances
Decreased appetite	Weight gain or loss
Increased respiratory rate, heart rate, cardiac output, and blood pressure	Increased risk for myocardial infarction and stroke
Increased metabolism and glucose use	Poor diabetes control, hypertension, fatigue, irritability, and decreased ability to concentrate
Depressed immune system	Increased risk for infection

- Standardized Screening Tools

- o   Life-changing events questionnaires (Holmes and Rahe scale to measure Life Change Units, Lazarus's Cognitive Appraisal)

Collaborative Care

- Nursing Care

- o   Reinforce teaching of stress-reduction strategies to clients.

- o   Cognitive techniques

  - ■   Cognitive reframing

    - □   Clients are helped to look at irrational cognitions (thoughts) in a more realistic light and to restructure those thoughts in a more positive way.

    - □   For example, a client may think he is "a terrible father to my daughter." A health professional using therapeutic communication techniques could help the person reframe that thought into a positive, such as, "I've made some bad mistakes as a parent, but I've learned from them and have improved my parenting skills."

- o   Behavioral techniques

  - ■   Relaxation techniques

    - □   Meditation includes formal meditation techniques, as well as prayer for those who believe in a higher power.

    - □   Guided imagery – Clients are guided through a series of images to promote relaxation. Images vary depending on the individual. For example, one client might imagine walking on a beach, while another client might imagine himself in a position of success.

- □ Breathing exercises are used to decrease rapid breathing and promote relaxation.

- □ Progressive muscle relaxation (PMR) – A person trained in this method can help clients attain complete relaxation within a few minutes of time.

- □ Physical exercise (yoga, walking, biking) causes release of endorphins that lower anxiety, promote relaxation, and have antidepressant effects.

- ■ Journal writing

  - □ Journaling has been shown to allow for a therapeutic release of stress.

  - □ This activity can help clients identify stressors and make specific plans to decrease stressors.

- ■ Priority restructuring

  - □ Clients learn to prioritize differently to reduce the number of stressors impacting them.

  - □ For example, a person who is under stress due to feeling overworked might delegate some tasks to others rather than doing them all herself.

- ■ Biofeedback

  - □ A nurse or other health professional trained in this method can assist clients to gain voluntary control of such autonomic functions as heart rate and blood pressure.

- ■ Assertiveness training

  - □ Clients learn to communicate in a more assertive manner in order to decrease psychological stressors.

  - □ For example, one technique teaches a client to assert his feelings by describing a situation or behavior that causes stress, stating his feelings about the behavior or situation, and then making a change. The client states, "When you keep telling me what to do, I feel angry and frustrated. I need to try making some of my own decisions."

- • Client Outcomes

  - ○ The client will verbalize stressors and ways to decrease exposure.

  - ○ The client will demonstrate appropriate relaxation techniques.

  - ○ The client will demonstrate assertive communication.

Ⓐ APPLICATION EXERCISES

Scenario: A client speaking to a nurse in a general medical clinic describes herself as feeling anxious, apprehensive, and tired all the time. She says she cannot understand why, since she is very happy. She recently moved to the area to start a new job for a large corporation. She purchased a new and much larger home for herself and her three children, ages 5, 8, and 12. The children transitioned to their new schools successfully and are making friends. The client's family and friends are all back in the previous city where she lived, but she has been so busy with work that she has not had time to telephone or write to them. The client states she has not been able to sleep and has lost weight in the 2 months since the move.

1. List the stressors that affect this client.

2. Which of this client's manifestations of increased stress reflects acute stress rather than prolonged stress?

   A. Weight loss
   B. Apprehension
   C. Fatigue
   D. Insomnia

3. A client says she is experiencing increased stress because her significant other "leaves the house in the evening, saying that he is going to work but I know he is not there." She also states that he "keeps nagging at my oldest son, which makes me mad, since he's my son, not his." Which of the following coping strategies might the nurse suggest for this client?

   A. Learn to reframe the situation.
   B. Use assertiveness techniques.
   C. Exercise regularly.
   D. Use guided imagery.

APPLICATION EXERCISES ANSWER KEY

Scenario: A client speaking to a nurse in a general medical clinic describes herself as feeling anxious, apprehensive, and tired all the time. She says she cannot understand why, since she is very happy. She recently moved to the area to start a new job for a large corporation. She purchased a new and much larger home for herself and her three children, ages 5, 8, and 12. The children transitioned to their new schools successfully and are making friends. The client's family and friends are all back in the previous city where she lived, but she has been so busy with work that she has not had time to telephone or write to them. The client states she has not been able to sleep and has lost weight in the 2 months since the move.

1. List the stressors that affect this client.

   Recent move

   Purchase and move into larger home

   Three children transferring to a different school

   Sudden decrease in support systems

   New job

   Lack of free time

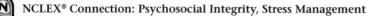 NCLEX® Connection: Psychosocial Integrity, Stress Management

2. Which of this client's manifestations of increased stress reflects acute stress rather than prolonged stress?

   A. Weight loss
   B. Apprehension
   C. Fatigue
   D. Insomnia

   Apprehension is a manifestation of acute stress. Prolonged stress leads to weight loss, fatigue, and insomnia.

   NCLEX® Connection: Psychosocial Integrity, Stress Management

3. A client says she is experiencing increased stress because her significant other "leaves the house in the evening, saying that he is going to work but I know he is not there." She also states that he "keeps nagging at my oldest son, which makes me mad, since he's my son, not his." Which of the following coping strategies might the nurse suggest for this client?

   A. Learn to reframe the situation.

   B. Use assertiveness techniques.

   C. Exercise regularly.

   D. Use guided imagery.

   Assertiveness techniques would help this client make her feelings known and request a change of behavior without using blaming or other negative communication. Reframing the situation is not appropriate because the stressor does not seem to be caused by irrational thoughts. Exercise and guided imagery might decrease the client's stress, but they would not change the situation.

   NCLEX® Connection: Psychosocial Integrity, Stress Management

UNIT 2	TRADITIONAL NONPHARMACOLOGIC THERAPIES
Chapter 9	Electroconvulsive Therapy

Overview

- Electroconvulsive therapy (ECT) is an alternative somatic treatment for mental health disorders.

- ECT delivers an electrical current that produces a grand mal seizure.

- The exact mechanism of ECT is still unknown and controversial. One theory suggests that ECT may enhance the effects of neurotransmitters (serotonin, dopamine, norepinephrine) in the brain.

Indications

- Severe Depression

  ○ Clients whose symptoms are not responsive to pharmacologic treatment

  ○ Clients for whom the risks of other treatments outweigh the risks of ECT, such as a client who is in her first trimester of pregnancy

  ○ Clients who are actively suicidal and for whom there is a need for rapid therapeutic response

- Certain types of schizophrenia that are less responsive to neuroleptic medications (catatonic schizophrenia, schizoaffective disorders)

- Acute Manic Episodes

  ○ ECT is used for clients who have bipolar disorder with rapid cycling (four or more episodes of acute mania within 1 year) and very destructive behavior. Both of these features tend to respond poorly to lithium therapy. These clients receive ECT and then a regimen of lithium therapy.

Contraindications

- There are no absolute contraindications for this therapy if it is deemed necessary to save/improve a client's life. However, the nurse should be aware that some clients may have medical conditions that place them at higher risk if ECT is used. These conditions include:

  ○ Recent myocardial infarction

  ○ History of cerebrovascular accident

- o Cerebrovascular malformation
- o Intracranial mass lesion
- Mental health conditions for which ECT has not been found useful include:
  - o Developmental disabilities
  - o Chemical dependence
  - o Personality disorders
  - o Situational depression

Client Outcomes

- The client is relieved of clinical manifestations of depression.
- The client is able to perform activities of daily living.

Nursing Actions

- Preparation of the Client
  - o The typical course of ECT treatment is three times a week for a total of six to 12 treatments.
  - o Use therapeutic communication prior to the procedure and throughout the course of ECT treatments.
  - o The provider discusses the procedure (including all risks and benefits, as well as a description of the procedure) with the client, and informed consent is obtained.
    - A guardian must give consent for ECT for a client who has been declared incompetent. Some clients who have been declared incompetent require a court order.
    - Some facilities require a separate informed consent for anesthesia, which would be obtained by an anesthesia provider.
    - A history and physical examination, including a neurological examination, electrocardiogram, and laboratory tests (complete blood count and other tests prescribed by the provider or per facility protocol) are obtained.

 View Media Supplement: Electroconvulsive Therapy (ECT) (Image)

  - o Medication management
    - Any medications that affect the client's seizure threshold must be decreased or discontinued several days before the ECT procedure.
    - MAOIs and lithium should be discontinued 2 weeks before the ECT procedure.
  - o Severe hypertension is controlled, since a short period of hypertension occurs immediately after the ECT procedure.

- o The nurse monitors the client's vital signs and mental status before and after the ECT procedure.

- o The nurse also asks the client and his family about their understanding and knowledge of the procedure and redirects the client to the provider for clarification as necessary.

- o An IV catheter is inserted and maintained until full recovery.

- o Thirty minutes prior to the beginning of the procedure, an IM injection of atropine sulfate or glycopyrrolate (Robinul) is given to decrease secretions and counteract any vagal stimulation.

- Ongoing Care

  - o ECT is administered early in the morning after the client has fasted for 8 to 12 hr.

  - o The client uses a bite guard to prevent trauma to the oral cavity.

  - o Electrodes are applied to the scalp, either unilaterally or bilaterally. The exact number and placement of electrodes is decided by the provider.

  - o The client is mechanically ventilated during the procedure and receives 100% oxygen.

  - o Ongoing cardiac monitoring is provided, including blood pressure, cardiac rate and rhythm, and oxygen saturation.

  - o An anesthesia provider administers a short-acting anesthetic, such as methohexital (Brevital) via IV bolus.

  - o A muscle relaxant, such as succinylcholine (Anectine), is then administered.

  - o A cuff is placed on one leg or arm to block the muscle relaxant so that seizure activity can be monitored in the limb distal to the cuff.

  - o The electrical stimulus is typically applied for 0.2 to 0.8 seconds. Seizure activity is monitored, and the duration of the seizure, which is usually 25 to 60 seconds, is documented.

  - o After seizure activity has ceased, the anesthetic is discontinued.

  - o The client is extubated and assisted to breathe voluntarily.

- Postprocedure Care

  - o When stable, the client is transferred to a recovery area where level of consciousness, cardiac status, vital signs, and oxygen saturation continue to be monitored.

  - o Position the client on his side to facilitate drainage and prevent aspiration.

  - o The client is usually awake and ready for transfer back to the mental health unit or other facility within 30 to 60 minutes after the procedure.

  - o During the recovery phase, orient the client frequently, because confusion and short-term memory loss are common during this time.

  - o Continue to monitor the client's vital signs as indicated and mental status for memory loss.

Complications

- Memory Loss and Confusion

  o Short-term memory loss, confusion, and disorientation may occur immediately following the procedure. Memory loss may persist for several weeks. Whether or not ECT causes permanent memory loss is controversial.

  o Nursing Actions

    ■ Provide frequent orientation.

    ■ Provide a safe environment to prevent injury.

    ■ Assist the client with personal hygiene as needed.

  o Client Education

    ■ Explain to clients and families that memory loss is typically short term.

    ■ Assist clients with memory during this period.

      □ Place a clock in the client's room.

      □ Label the client's room location.

- Headache, muscle soreness, and nausea can occur during and following the immediate recovery period.

  o Nursing Actions

    ■ Observe clients to determine the degree of discomfort.

    ■ Administer antiemetic and analgesic medications as needed.

  o Client Education

    ■ Explain the reason for the clinical manifestations to clients.

    ■ Encourage clients to contact the nurse regarding these clinical manifestations.

Ⓐ APPLICATION EXERCISES

Scenario: A client who has major depression and has not responded to antidepressant medications is admitted to an acute care mental health facility for ECT. The client is voluntarily receiving ECT; however, the client and his family have concerns about the treatment.

1. List the care to be provided for the client and the client's family.

2. The client's family says, "We were already told that people are really confused after ECT. Besides that, what other problems should we expect after the procedure?" How should the nurse reply?

3. Which of the following is a possible indication for ECT?

    A. Borderline personality disorder
    B. Suicidal ideation caused by a recent loss
    C. Catatonic schizophrenia
    D. A developmental disability

APPLICATION EXERCISES ANSWER KEY

Scenario: A client who has major depression and has not responded to antidepressant medications is admitted to an acute care mental health facility for ECT. The client is voluntarily receiving ECT; however, the client and his family have concerns about the treatment.

1. List the care to be provided for the client and the client's family.

    Review the client's medical history.

    Collaborate with the mental health care provider about the specific instructions for the ECT procedure as it applies to this client.

    Explain the adverse reactions of the procedure to the client and the family in short, easy-to-understand statements.

    Be consistent when explaining procedures.

    Reinforce to the client and the family about safety precautions and maintenance of self-care needs.

    Listen to the client's and the family's concerns and fears.

    Check if the client has withheld any medications per instructions from the provider.

    Help the client and the family to make and adhere to schedules for future ECT appointments.

 NCLEX® Connection: Reduction of Risk Potential, Potential for Complications of Diagnostic Tests/Treatments/Procedure

2. The client's family says, "We were already told that people are really confused after ECT. Besides that, what other problems should we expect after the procedure?" How should the nurse reply?

    It is not uncommon for clients who receive ECT to develop a headache, muscle soreness, or nausea during and following the immediate recovery period.

 NCLEX® Connection: Reduction of Risk Potential, Potential for Complications of Diagnostic Tests/Treatments/Procedure

3. Which of the following is a possible indication for ECT?

    A. Borderline personality disorder

    B. Suicidal ideation caused by a recent loss

    C. Catatonic schizophrenia

    D. A developmental disability

    The client who has catatonic schizophrenia and is unresponsive to neuroleptic medications is a possible candidate for ECT. Clients who are not usually good candidates for ECT include those with personality disorders, situational depression, chemical dependency, or a developmental disability.

Ⓝ NCLEX® Connection: Reduction of Risk Potential, Potential for Complications of Diagnostic Tests/Treatments/Procedure

UNIT 3: PSYCHOBIOLOGIC DISORDERS

- Anxiety Disorders
- Depression
- Bipolar Disorders
- Schizophrenia
- Personality Disorders
- Cognitive Disorders
- Substance and Other Dependencies
- Eating Disorders

NCLEX® CONNECTIONS

When reviewing the chapters in this section, keep in mind the relevant sections of the NCLEX® outline, in particular:

CLIENT NEEDS: PSYCHOSOCIAL INTEGRITY

Relevant topics/tasks include:
- Behavioral Management
  - Explore cause of client behavior.
- Chemical and Other Dependencies
  - Plan and provide care to client experiencing substance-related withdrawal or toxicity.
- Coping Mechanisms
  - Identify client use of effective and ineffective coping mechanisms.
- Mental Health Concepts
  - Recognize client symptoms of relapse.

CLIENT NEEDS: PHARMACOLOGICAL THERAPIES

Relevant topics/tasks include:
- Adverse Effects/Contraindications/Side Effects/Interactions
  - Monitor and document client side effects to medications.
- Expected Actions/Outcomes
  - Apply knowledge of pathophysiology when addressing client pharmacological agents.
- Medication Administration
  - Identify client need for PRN medications.

UNIT 3	PSYCHOBIOLOGIC DISORDERS
Chapter 10	Anxiety Disorders

Overview

- Anxiety is a response to stress. Higher levels of anxiety result in behavior changes. Anxiety tends to be persistent and is often disabling.

- Anxiety levels can be mild (restlessness, increased motivation, irritability), moderate (agitation, muscle tightness), severe (inability to function, ritualistic behavior, unresponsive), or panic (distorted perception or hallucinations, loss of rational thought, immobility).

- The various anxiety disorders recognized and defined by the DSM-IV-TR include:

  ○ Panic disorder – Clients experience recurrent panic attacks.

  ○ Phobias – Clients fear a specific object or situation to an unreasonable level.

  ○ Obsessive compulsive disorder (OCD) – Clients have intrusive thoughts of unrealistic obsessions and try to control these thoughts with compulsive behaviors (repetitive cleaning of a particular object, constantly performing hand hygiene).

  ○ Generalized anxiety disorder (GAD) – Clients exhibit uncontrollable, excessive worry for more than 6 months.

  ○ Stress-related disorders include:

    ■ Acute stress disorder – Exposure to a traumatic event causes numbing, detachment, and amnesia about the event for not more than four weeks following the event.

    ■ Posttraumatic stress disorder (PTSD) – Exposure to a traumatic event causes intense fear, horror, flashbacks, feelings of detachment and foreboding, restricted affect, and impairment for longer than one month after the event. Symptoms may last for years.

- Defense mechanisms are cognitive distortions used to deal with stress, and their use is common in individuals with anxiety disorders. Commonly used defense mechanisms include displacement, undoing, reaction formation, intellectualization, isolation, and repression.

Data Collection

- Risk Factors

  - Except for OCD, which has equal prevalence in men and women, anxiety disorders are much more likely to occur in women.

  - Exposure to a traumatic event or experience (military combat, threat of death of a loved one) can precipitate an anxiety disorder.

  - Experiencing smells or sounds attached to a traumatic event can trigger a panic attack

  - Anxiety can be due to an acute medical condition, such as pulmonary embolism. It is important that clinical findings of anxiety be evaluated in the appropriate medical facility to rule out a physical cause.

  - Substance-induced anxiety can be related to current use of a chemical substance or to withdrawal symptoms from a substance, such as alcohol.

- Subjective and Objective Data

  - Panic disorder

    - Episodes typically last 15 to 30 min.

    - Four or more of the following clinical manifestations are present:

      - Palpitations
      - Shortness of breath
      - Choking or smothering sensation
      - Chest pain
      - Nausea
      - Feelings of depersonalization
      - Fear of dying or insanity
      - Chills or hot flashes

    - Clients may experience behavior changes and/or persistent worries about when the next attack will occur.

    - Clients may begin to experience agoraphobia due to a fear of being in places where previous panic attacks occurred. For example, if previous attacks occurred while driving, the client may stop driving. If attacks continue while walking or taking alternative transportation, the client may remain at home.

  - Phobias

    - Social phobia – Clients have a fear of embarrassment, are unable to perform in front of others, have a dread of social situations, believe that others are judging them negatively, and have impaired relationships.

    - Agoraphobia – Clients avoid being outside and have an impaired ability to work or perform duties.

- Specific phobias
  - Clients have a fear of specific objects (spiders, snakes, strangers).
  - Clients have a fear of specific experiences (flying, being in the dark, riding in an elevator, being in an enclosed space).
- Obsessive compulsive disorder (OCD)
  - Clients who engage in constant ritualistic behaviors may have difficulty meeting self-care needs (personal hygiene, grooming, nutrition, fluid intake, elimination, or sleep).
  - If rituals include performing constant hand hygiene, skin damage and infection may occur.
- Generalized anxiety disorder (GAD)
  - GAD causes significant impairment in one or more areas of functioning, such as work-related duties.
  - At least three of the following clinical manifestations are present:
    - Fatigue
    - Restlessness
    - Problems with concentration
    - Irritability
    - Increased muscle tension
    - Sleep disturbances
- Stress-related disorders

ACUTE STRESS DISORDER	PTSD
Precipitating event	
<ul><li>In both disorders, clients witness or experience an actual event that threatens severe injury or death to them or others.</li><li>Clients respond with fear, helplessness, or horror to the event.</li></ul>	
First symptoms	
• Clinical findings occur within 4 weeks of the traumatic event.	• The onset of clinical findings is delayed at least 3 months from the precipitating event, and onset may not occur until years afterward.
Duration	

• Clinical findings last from 2 days to 4 weeks.	• Clinical findings last more than 1 month.
	  ○ Acute PTSD – Duration less than 3 months
	  ○ Chronic PTSD – Duration more than 3 months

ACUTE STRESS DISORDER	PTSD
Re-experience of the event	

• Clients persistently re-experience the event through:
  ○ Distress when reminded of the event
  ○ Dreams or images
  ○ Reliving through flashbacks
	• Clients persistently re-experience the event through:
	  ○ Recurrent, intrusive recollection of the event
	  ○ Dreams or images
	  ○ Reliving through flashbacks, illusions, or hallucinations

Clinical findings	
• Dissociative symptoms, such as amnesia of the trauma event, absent emotional response, decreased awareness of surroundings, and depersonalization • Clinical findings of severe anxiety, such as irritability and sleep disturbance	• Clinical findings of increased arousal, such as irritability, difficulty with concentration, and sleep disturbance • Avoidance of stimuli associated with trauma, such as avoiding people and inability to show feelings

- Standardized Screening Tools
  - Hamilton Rating Scale for Anxiety
  - Modified Spielberger State Anxiety Scale

Collaborative Care

- Nursing Care
  - Provide a structured interview to keep clients focused on the present.
  - Provide safety and comfort to clients during the crisis period of these disorders, as clients with severe- to panic-level anxiety are unable to problem-solve and focus. Do not reinforce teaching at this time.
  - Remain with clients during the worst of the anxiety to provide reassurance.
  - Provide a safe environment for other clients and staff.
  - Provide milieu therapy that employs the following:
    - A structured environment for physical safety and predictability
    - Monitoring for, and protection from, self-harm
    - Daily activities that encourage clients to share and be cooperative
    - Use of therapeutic communication skills, such as open-ended questions, to help clients express feelings of anxiety and to validate and acknowledge those feelings
    - Client participation in decision-making regarding care

- ○ Encourage clients with mild to moderate anxiety to use relaxation techniques as needed for symptoms of pain, muscle tension, and feelings of anxiety.

- ○ Instill hope for positive outcomes (but avoid false reassurance).

- ○ Enhance client self-esteem by encouraging positive statements and discussing past achievements.

- ○ Assist clients to identify defense mechanisms that interfere with recovery.

- ○ Postpone reinforcing client education until after acute anxiety subsides. Clients experiencing a panic attack or severe anxiety are unable to concentrate or learn.

- ○ Specific therapies include:

  - ■ Cognitive reframing – The anxiety response can be decreased by changing cognitive distortions. This therapy assists clients to identify negative thoughts that produce anxiety, examine the cause, and develop supportive ideas that replace negative self-talk.

  - ■ Behavioral therapies teach clients ways to decrease anxiety or avoidant behavior and allow an opportunity to practice techniques.

    - □ Relaxation training can be used to control pain, tension, and anxiety.

    - □ Modeling allows clients to see a demonstration of appropriate behavior in a stressful situation. The goal of therapy is that clients will be able to imitate the behavior.

    - □ Systematic desensitization begins with mastering of relaxation techniques. Then, clients are exposed to increasing levels of an anxiety-producing stimulus (either imagined or real) and use relaxation to overcome the resulting anxiety. The goal of therapy is that clients will be able to tolerate a greater and greater level of the stimulus until anxiety no longer interferes with functioning.

    - □ Flooding involves exposing clients to a great deal of an undesirable stimulus in an attempt to turn off the anxiety response.

    - □ Response prevention focuses on preventing clients from performing a compulsive behavior with the intent that anxiety will diminish.

    - □ Thought-stopping teaches clients to say "stop" when negative thoughts or compulsive behaviors arise and to substitute a positive thought. The goal of therapy is that with time clients use the command silently.

  - ■ Eye movement desensitization therapy (EMDR) – Combines cognitive-behavioral therapy with eye movements or rhythmic sound stimulation. The goal of this treatment is to unfreeze fragments or trauma so they can be integrated back into memory and processed.

  - ■ Group and family therapy for clients with PTSD

- Medications

  o Use antidepressants (sertraline [Zoloft], amitriptyline [Elavil]), sedative hypnotic anxiolytics (diazepam [Valium]), serotonin norepinephrine reuptake inhibitors (venlafaxine [Effexor]), and nonbarbiturate anxiolytics (buspirone [BuSpar]) to manage anxiety.

  o Other medications to use to treat anxiety disorders include beta blockers, antihistamines, and anticonvulsants as mood stabilizers for clients who experience anxiety. Use mirtazapine (Remeron), a serotonin norepinephrine disinhibitor, to help clients rest when panic attacks occur during sleep.

- Care After Discharge

  o Client education

    ■ Reinforce to clients regarding identification of clinical manifestations of anxiety.

    ■ Instruct clients to notify the provider of worsening symptoms and to not adjust medication dosages. Warn clients against stopping or increasing medication without consultation with the provider.

    ■ Assist clients to evaluate coping mechanisms that work and do not work for controlling the anxiety, and assist clients to learn new methods. Use of alternative stress relief and coping mechanisms can increase medication effectiveness and decrease the need for medication in most cases.

Client Outcomes

- The client will verbalize decreased feelings of anxiety.

- The client will be rested upon awakening.

- The client will develop realistic goals for the future.

- The client will regularly attend a support group.

- The client will demonstrate appropriate use of relaxation techniques.

Ⓐ **APPLICATION EXERCISES**

1. When collecting data from a client who states that she has been dealing with constant anxiety for the past few weeks, the nurse should use which of the following communication techniques? (Select all that apply.)

    _____ Ask open-ended questions.

    _____ Provide reassurance.

    _____ Discuss the client's past achievements.

    _____ Offer advice about how to reduce anxiety.

    _____ Invite the client to participate in decision-making.

2. A client being evaluated in her provider's office tells the nurse, "I remove my old makeup and apply new makeup every hour or so because I look horrible." The nurse should understand that this behavior is characteristic of which of the following disorders?

    A. Generalized anxiety disorder (GAD)

    B. Agoraphobia

    C. Obsessive-compulsive disorder (OCD)

    D. Post-traumatic stress disorder (PTSD)

3. An appropriate nursing intervention for a client having a panic attack is to

    A. suggest relaxation techniques for the client.

    B. show the client how to change her behavior.

    C. distract the client with a television show.

    D. stay with the client and speak quietly.

4. Match the specific anxiety disorder with its characteristics.

_____ Obsessive-compulsive disorder	A. Traumatic event causing symptoms for months after the event takes place
_____ Panic disorder	B. Exposure to a traumatic event, resulting in numbing, detachment, and amnesia about the event for up to 4 weeks
_____ Acute stress disorder	C. Fear of speaking with or interacting with others
_____ Agoraphobia	D. Clinical findings including chest pain, palpitations, feelings of impending doom
_____ Social phobia	E. Fear of being out in open spaces
_____ Post-traumatic stress disorder	F. Ritualistic compulsions and recurrent thoughts

APPLICATION EXERCISES ANSWER KEY

1. When collecting data from a client who states that she has been dealing with constant anxiety for the past few weeks, the nurse should use which of the following communication techniques? (Select all that apply.)

    X   **Ask open-ended questions.**

    _____ Provide reassurance.

    X   **Discuss the client's past achievements.**

    _____ Offer advice about how to reduce anxiety.

    X   **Invite the client to participate in decision-making.**

    Open-ended questions allow the client to tell the nurse about her anxiety. Talking about past achievements and encouraging input into care decisions help enhance the client's self-esteem. Providing reassurance and offering advice are examples of nontherapeutic communication that dismiss the client's concerns.

 NCLEX® Connection: Psychosocial Integrity, Therapeutic Communication

2. A client being evaluated in her provider's office tells the nurse, "I remove my old makeup and apply new makeup every hour or so because I look horrible." The nurse should understand that this behavior is characteristic of which of the following disorders?

    A. Generalized anxiety disorder (GAD)

    B. Agoraphobia

    C. Obsessive-compulsive disorder (OCD)

    D. Post-traumatic stress disorder (PTSD)

    OCD is characterized by repetitive, unreasonable behavior used to reduce anxiety, such as the hourly reapplication of makeup. GAD is characterized by excessive worry over multiple concerns for more than 6 months. With agoraphobia, the client fears being outdoors. PTSD causes repeated re-experiencing of a traumatic event.

 NCLEX® Connection: Psychosocial Integrity, Mental Health Concepts

3. An appropriate nursing intervention for a client having a panic attack is to

    A. suggest relaxation techniques for the client.

    B. show the client how to change her behavior.

    C. distract the client with a television show.

    D. stay with the client and speak quietly.

    During a panic attack, the client is unable to think about anything except her symptoms. The nurse should stay with her, as the client will not be distractible and cannot concentrate on learning new material. The nurse should postpone other interventions until after the attack.

 NCLEX® Connection: Psychosocial Integrity, Crisis Intervention

4. Match the specific anxiety disorder with its characteristics.

F	Obsessive-compulsive disorder	A. Traumatic event causing symptoms for months after the event takes place
D	Panic disorder	B. Exposure to a traumatic event, resulting in numbing, detachment, and amnesia about the event for up to 4 weeks
B	Acute stress disorder	C. Fear of speaking with or interacting with others
E	Agoraphobia	
C	Social phobia	D. Clinical findings including chest pain, palpitations, feelings of impending doom
A	Post-traumatic stress disorder	E. Fear of being out in open spaces
		F. Ritualistic compulsions and recurrent thoughts

 NCLEX® Connection: Psychosocial Integrity, Mental Health Concepts

UNIT 3	PSYCHOBIOLOGIC DISORDERS
Chapter 11	Depression

Overview

- Depression is a mood (affective) disorder that is a widespread issue, ranking high among causes of disability.

- Depression may be comorbid with the following:

  o Anxiety disorders

    ▪ These disorders are comorbid with 70% of major depressive disorders, the combination of which makes a client's prognosis poorer, with a higher risk for suicide and disability.

  o Schizophrenia

  o Substance abuse

    ▪ Clients often abuse substances in order to relieve symptoms and/or self-treat mental health disorders.

  o Eating disorders

  o Personality disorders

- A client with depression may be at risk for suicide, especially if the client has a family or personal history of suicide attempts, comorbid anxiety disorder or panic attacks, comorbid substance abuse or psychosis, poor self-esteem, a lack of social support, or a chronic medical condition.

- Depressive disorders recognized and defined by the DSM-IV-TR include:

  o Major depressive disorder (MDD) is a single episode or recurrent episodes of unipolar depression (not associated with mood swings from major depression to mania) resulting in a significant change in a client's normal functioning (social, occupational, self-care) accompanied by at least five of the following specific clinical manifestations, which must occur almost every day for a minimum of 2 weeks, and last most of the day:

    ▪ Depressed mood

    ▪ Difficulty sleeping or excessive sleeping

    ▪ Indecisiveness

    ▪ Decreased ability to concentrate

    ▪ Suicidal ideation

- Increase or decrease in motor activity

- Inability to feel pleasure

- Increase or decrease in weight of more than 5% of total body weight over one month

○ MDD may be further diagnosed in the DSM-IV-TR with a more specific classification (specifier), including:

- Psychotic features – The presence of auditory hallucinations (voices telling the client she is sinful) or the presence of delusions (client thinking that she has a fatal disease)

- Atypical features – Changes in appetite or weight gain, and excessive daytime sleepiness

- Postpartum onset – A depressive episode that begins within 4 weeks of childbirth (known as postpartum depression) and may include delusions, which may put the newborn infant at high risk of being harmed by the mother

- Seasonal characteristics – Seasonal affective disorder (SAD), which occurs during winter and may be treated with light therapy

- Chronic features – A depressive episode that lasts more than 2 years

○ Dysthymic disorder is a milder, more chronic form of depression that usually has an early onset, such as in childhood or adolescence, and lasts at least 2 years in length for adults (1 year in length for children). Dysthymic disorder contains at least three clinical findings of depression and may, later in life, become major depressive disorder. This disorder differs from major depression in that the clinical manifestations are less severe.

○ Care of a client with MDD will mirror the phase of the disease that the client is experiencing:

PHASE	CHARACTERISTICS	TREATMENT
Acute	Severe clinical findings of depression	• Treatment is generally 6 to 12 weeks in duration • Hospitalization may be required. • Reduction of depressive symptoms is the goal of treatment. • Suicide potential is determined and safety precautions are implemented. • One-to-one observation may be indicated.
Maintenance	Increased ability to function	• Treatment is generally 4 to 9 months in duration • Relapse prevention through education, medication therapy, and psychotherapy is the goal of treatment.
Continuation	Remission of clinical findings	• This phase may last for years. • Prevention of future depressive episodes is the goal of treatment.

Data Collection

- Risk Factors

    o Family history and a previous personal history of depression are the most significant risk factors.

    o Depressive disorders are twice as common in females between the ages of 15 and 40 as in males.

    o Depression is very common among clients over age 65, but the disorder is more difficult to recognize in the older adult client and may go untreated. It is important to differentiate between early dementia and depression. Some clinical manifestations of depression that may look like dementia are memory loss, confusion, and behavioral problems (social isolation, agitation). Clients may seek health care for somatic symptoms that are manifestations of untreated depression.

    o A neurotransmitter deficiency (serotonin deficiency) that affects mood, sexual behavior, sleep cycles, hunger, and pain perception can be a risk factor for depression.

    o Other risk factors include:

      ▪ Stressful life events

      ▪ Presence of a medical illness

      ▪ Being a female in the postpartum period

      ▪ Poor social support network

      ▪ Comorbid substance abuse

    o Depression occurs throughout all groups of people. There are no specific risk factors for ethnicity, education, income, or marital status.

    o Depression may be the primary disorder, or it may be a response to another physical or mental health disorder.

- Subjective Data

    o Anergia (lack of energy)

    o Anhedonia (lack of pleasure in normal activities)

    o Anxiety

    o Reports of sluggishness (most common) or feeling unable to relax and sit still

    o Vegetative findings, which include a change in eating patterns (usually anorexia in MDD, and increased intake in dysthymia), change in bowel habits (usually constipation), sleep disturbances, and decreased interest in sexual activity

    o Somatic reports (fatigue, gastrointestinal symptoms, pain)

- Objective Data

  o Physical assessment findings

    - Appears sad with a blunted affect

    - Poor grooming and lack of hygiene

    - Psychomotor retardation (slowed physical movement, slumped posture) is more common, but psychomotor agitation (restlessness, pacing, finger tapping) can also occur.

    - Shows little or no effort to interact, becoming socially isolated

    - Slowed speech, decreased verbalization, and delayed response – The client may seem too tired even to speak.

- Standardized Screening Tools

  o Hamilton Depression Scale

  o Beck Depression Inventory

   o Geriatric Depression Scale (short form)

  o Zung Self-Rating Depression Scale

  o A confidential screening tool (http://www.depression-screening.org)

Collaborative Care

- Nursing Care

  o Milieu therapy

    - Self-care – Monitor the client's ability to perform activities of daily living and encourage independence as much as possible. Encourage participation in treatment therapy and decision-making process.

    - Communication

      □ Relate therapeutically to clients who are unable or unwilling to communicate.

      □ Make time to be with clients, even if clients do not speak.

      □ Make observations rather than asking direct questions, which may cause anxiety in the client. For example, the nurse might say, "I noticed that you attended the unit group meeting today," rather than asking, "Did you enjoy the group meeting?" Give directions in simple, concrete sentences because the client with depression may have difficulty focusing on and comprehending long sentences.

      □ Give the client sufficient time to respond when holding a conversation; the client's response time may be greatly slowed.

     - Maintenance of a safe environment

View Media Supplement: Understanding Major Depression (Video)

- Medications

  o Antidepressants

    ■ Client teaching for all antidepressants

      □ Tell clients not to discontinue medication suddenly.

      □ Inform clients that medications may take 1 to 3 weeks for therapeutic effects for initial response with up to 2 months for maximal response.

      □ Instruct clients to avoid hazardous activities (driving, operating heavy equipment/machinery).

MEDICATION CLASSIFICATION/EXAMPLE	NURSING CONSIDERATIONS/CLIENT EDUCATION
Selective serotonin reuptake inhibitors (SSRIs) • Citalopram (Celexa) • Fluoxetine (Prozac) • Sertraline (Zoloft)	• Inform clients that side effects may include nausea, headache, and CNS stimulation (agitation, insomnia, anxiety). • Tell clients that sexual dysfunction may occur. Notify the provider if effects are intolerable. • Instruct clients to follow healthy diet, as weight gain can occur with long-term use.
Tricyclic antidepressants • Amitriptyline (Elavil)	• Advise clients to change positions slowly to minimize dizziness from orthostatic hypotension.
Monoamine Oxidase Inhibitors (MAOIs) • Phenelzine (Nardil)	• Advise clients to chew sugarless gum, eat foods high in fiber, and increase fluid intake to 2 to 3 L/day from food and beverage sources to minimize anticholinergic effects. • Advise clients to avoid foods with tyramine (ripe avocados or figs, fermented or smoked meats, liver, dried or cured fish, most cheeses, some beer and wine, protein dietary supplements). Combinations of this medication and the above foods can cause hypertensive crisis and even death.

Sedative hypnotic anxiolytics (Benzodiazepines)
• Diazepam (Valium)
• Lorazepam (Ativan)
	• Instruct clients to:
	  o Watch for CNS depression (sedation, lightheadedness, ataxia, decreased cognitive function).
	  o Avoid the use of other CNS depressants (alcohol).
	  o Avoid hazardous activities (driving, operating heavy equipment/machinery).
	  o Avoid caffeine, which interferes with the desired effects of the medication.

Serotonin norepinephrine reuptake inhibitors • Venlafaxine (Effexor)	• Tell clients side effects include nausea, weight gain, and sexual dysfunction.
Nonbarbiturate anxiolytics • Buspirone (BuSpar)	• Inform clients that onset of therapeutic effects may take 2 to 4 weeks.

- Interdisciplinary Care

  o Psychotherapy by a trained therapist may include individual cognitive-behavioral therapy, group therapy, and family therapy. These therapies are intended to assist clients with:

    ▪ Problem solving

    ▪ Increasing coping abilities

    ▪ Changing negative thinking to positive

    ▪ Increasing self-esteem

    ▪ Assertiveness training

    ▪ Using available community resources

- Alternative or Complementary Therapies

  o St. John's Wort – The plant product (*Hypericum perforatum*), not regulated by the United States FDA, is taken by some individuals to relieve symptoms of mild depression.

    ▪ Client Education

      □ Inform clients that side effects include photosensitivity, skin rash, rapid heart rate, gastrointestinal distress, and abdominal pain.

      □ Instruct clients to inform the provider of use of St. John's Wort. St. John's Wort can increase or reduce levels of some medications if taken concurrently.

      □ Potentially fatal serotonin syndrome can result if St. John's Wort is taken with SSRIs, MAOIs, atypical antidepressants, and tricyclic antidepressants.

  o Light therapy – A first-line treatment for seasonal affective disorder (SAD), light therapy inhibits nocturnal secretion of melatonin.

    ▪ Exposure of the face to 10,000-lux light box 30 minutes a day, once or in two divided doses

- Therapeutic Procedures

  o Electroconvulsive therapy (ECT) can be useful for some clients with depression.

    ▪ Nursing Actions

      □ A specially trained nurse is responsible for monitoring the client before and after this therapy.

      □ Ensure clients have been observed for cardiovascular disease, neuromuscular disorders, and complicated pregnancy prior to beginning this treatment.

  o Transcranial magnetic stimulation (TMS) is a new therapy using electromagnetic stimulation of the brain; it may be helpful for depression that is resistant to other forms of treatment.

  o Vagus nerve stimulation (VNS therapy system) is an implanted device that stimulates the vagus nerve. It can be used for clients who have depression that is resistant to at least four antidepressant medications.

- Care After Discharge
  - Continuation phase followed by maintenance phase
    - Client Education
      - Review clinical manifestations of depression with clients and family members in order to identify relapse.
      - Reinforce intended effects and potential side effects of medication.
      - Explain the benefits of adherence to therapy.
      - Encourage regular exercise – Thirty minutes of exercise daily for three to five days each week improves clinical manifestations of depression and may help to prevent relapse. Even shorter intervals of exercise are helpful.
- Client Outcomes
  - The client will express increase in mood.
  - The client will adhere to the medication regimen.
  - The client will remain safe and notify the provider of any thoughts of suicide.

(A) **APPLICATION EXERCISES**

> **Scenario:** A 35-year-old female client is newly admitted to an acute-care mental health facility for her third episode of major depressive disorder. A teacher currently on medical leave, she lives at home with her husband and their two school-age children, but she has stopped cooking, doing housework, and grooming herself or the children during the past three weeks. She says she lacks the energy to do anything and has a poor appetite with a 5-lb weight loss, constipation, and an inability to sleep more than 5 hr each night (wakes up early and cannot get back to sleep). During the admission interview, she says to the nurse, "It would be better for my family if I just wasn't around ever again. I'm no good for them anymore, and I have no control over any part of my life."

1. Which of the following are risk factors for depression for this client? (Select all that apply.)

    _____ Age

    _____ Having two school-age children

    _____ History of depressive episodes

    _____ Being married

    _____ Occupation

2. The client is prescribed the SSRI paroxetine (Paxil) but wants to continue taking St. John's Wort. What should the nurse tell the client and spouse about taking this medication concurrently with St. John's Wort?

3. The client's husband asks the nurse, "How long will it be before we see if this new antidepressant medication is really going to work?" What should the nurse tell the client's spouse?

4. Which of the following interventions is the highest priority in managing this client's care?

    A. Placing the client on one-to-one observation

    B. Assisting the client to perform morning care

    C. Encouraging the client to participate in unit activities

    D. Suggesting that the client begin a regular exercise program

---

5. A nurse is interviewing a 25-year-old client diagnosed with dysthymia. Which of the following findings should the nurse expect?

    A. There are wide fluctuations in mood.

    B. There is no evidence of suicidal ideation.

    C. The symptoms last for at least two years.

    D. There is an inflated sense of self-esteem.

(A) APPLICATION EXERCISES ANSWER KEY

Scenario: A 35-year-old female client is newly admitted to an acute-care mental health facility for her third episode of major depressive disorder. A teacher currently on medical leave, she lives at home with her husband and their two school-age children, but she has stopped cooking, doing housework, and grooming herself or the children during the past 3 weeks. She says she lacks the energy to do anything and has a poor appetite with a 5-lb weight loss, constipation, and an inability to sleep more than 5 hr each night (wakes up early and cannot get back to sleep). During the admission interview, she says to the nurse, "It would be better for my family if I just wasn't around ever again. I'm no good for them anymore, and I have no control over any part of my life."

1. Which of the following are risk factors for depression for this client? (Select all that apply.)

   __X__ **Age**

   _____ Having two school-age children

   __X__ **History of depressive episodes**

   _____ Being married

   _____ Occupation

   Depression is most common between the ages of 15 and 40. A prior depressive episode places this client at risk for another episode. Having two small children, being a teacher, and being married are not risk factors for depression.

   (N) NCLEX® Connection: Psychosocial Integrity, Crisis Intervention

2. The client is prescribed the SSRI paroxetine (Paxil) but wants to continue taking St. John's Wort. What should the nurse tell the client and spouse about taking this medication concurrently with St. John's Wort?

   Combining any SSRI antidepressant with St. John's Wort can cause serotonin syndrome, a serious condition that includes high fever, hypertension, and delirium. The client should not continue to take St. John's Wort if prescribed paroxetine. Instruct client to notify the provider of all medications, including over-the-counter medications.

   (N) NCLEX® Connection: Pharmacological Therapies, Adverse Effects/Contraindications/Side Effects/Interactions

3. The client's husband asks the nurse, "How long will it be before we see if this new antidepressant medication is really going to work?" What should the nurse tell the client's spouse?

   The medication may take 1 to 3 weeks for an initial therapeutic response and up to 2 months for maximal response.

   (N) NCLEX® Connection: Pharmacological Therapies, Expected Actions/Outcomes

4. Which of the following interventions is the highest priority in managing this client's care?

   A. Placing the client on one-to-one observation

   B. Assisting the client to perform morning care

   C. Encouraging the client to participate in unit activities

   D. Suggesting that the client begin a regular exercise program

   The greatest risk to the client is self-injury. Therefore, the highest priority intervention is placing the client on one-to-one observation. Assisting her to perform morning care, encouraging her to participate in unit activities, and promoting exercise are all important interventions, but they are not the highest priority.

 NCLEX® Connection: Psychosocial Integrity, Crisis Intervention

5. A nurse is interviewing a 25-year-old client diagnosed with dysthymia. Which of the following findings should the nurse expect?

   A. There are wide fluctuations in mood.

   B. There is no evidence of suicidal ideation.

   C. The symptoms last for at least two years.

   D. There is an inflated sense of self-esteem.

   Symptoms of dysthymia persist for at least two years in adults and are usually less severe than with major depressive episode. Wide fluctuations in mood occur with bipolar disorders, but not with dysthymia. Suicidal ideation may occur in clients with dysthymia. A decreased, rather than inflated, sense of self-esteem is associated with dysthymia.

 NCLEX® Connection: Psychosocial Integrity, Mental Health Concepts

UNIT 3   PSYCHOBIOLOGIC DISORDERS

Chapter 12   Bipolar Disorders

Overview

- Bipolar disorders are mood disorders with recurrent episodes of depression and mania.

- Bipolar disorders usually emerge in late adolescence and early adulthood but can be diagnosed in the school-age child, as well. Because the side effects of medication and bipolar disorder clinical manifestations can mimic the symptoms of attention deficit hyperactivity disorder (ADHD), children are not usually diagnosed until after the age of seven.

- Periods of normal functioning alternate with periods of illness, though some clients are not able to maintain full occupational and social functioning.

- Psychotic, paranoid, and/or bizarre behavior may be seen during periods of mania.

- Care of clients with bipolar disorder will mirror the phase of the disease that the client is experiencing:

PHASE	CHARACTERISTICS	TREATMENT
Acute	Acute mania	<ul><li>Treatment is generally 6 to 12 weeks in duration.</li><li>Hospitalization may be required.</li><li>Reduction of mania symptoms is the goal of treatment.</li><li>Risk of harm to self or others is determined.</li><li>One-to-one supervision may be indicated.</li></ul>
Maintenance	Increased ability to function	<ul><li>Treatment is generally 4 to 9 months in duration.</li><li>Relapse prevention through education, medication therapy, and psychotherapy is the goal of treatment.</li></ul>
Continuation	Remission of symptoms	<ul><li>Treatment generally continues throughout the client's lifetime.</li><li>Prevention of future manic episodes is the goal of treatment.</li></ul>

- Behaviors shown with bipolar disorders include:

  o Mania – An abnormally elevated mood, which may also be described as expansive or irritable; usually requires inpatient treatment. (See the data collection section in this chapter for specific clinical findings.)

- o Hypomania – A less severe episode of mania that lasts at least 4 days accompanied by three to four clinical findings of mania. Hospitalization, however, is not required, and the client with hypomania is less impaired.

- o Mixed episode – A manic episode and an episode of major depression experienced by the client simultaneously. The client has marked impairment in functioning and may require admission to an acute care mental health facility to prevent self-harm or other-directed violence.

- o Rapid cycling – Four or more episodes of acute mania within 1 year.

- The various bipolar disorders recognized and defined by the DSM-IV-TR include the following:

  - o Bipolar I disorder – The client has at least one episode of mania alternating with major depression.

  - o Bipolar II disorder – The client has one or more hypomanic episodes alternating with major depressive episodes. Bipolar II differs from bipolar I in that clients do not have manic phases in bipolar II.

  - o Cyclothymia – The client has at least 2 years of repeated hypomanic episodes alternating with minor depressive episodes.

- The following comorbidities are associated with bipolar disorder:

  - o Substance abuse

    - ▪ The client with substance abuse issues tends to experience more rapid cycling of mania than do clients who are not abusing.

    - ▪ Substance use is often used as a means of self-medication. It can have a direct impact on the onset of a mental health disorder, especially if a client is predisposed.

  - o Anxiety disorders

  - o Eating disorders

  - o ADHD

Data Collection

- Risk Factors

  - o Physical illness, such as delirium due to a head injury

  - o Substance abuse, such as cocaine or methamphetamine overdose

- Relapse

  - o Use of substances (alcohol, drugs of abuse, caffeine) can lead to an episode of mania.

  - o Sleep disturbances may come before, be associated with, or be brought on by an episode of mania.

- Subjective and Objective Data

BIPOLAR DISORDER CLINICAL MANIFESTATIONS	
MANIC CHARACTERISTICS	DEPRESSIVE CHARACTERISTICS
<ul><li>Persistent elevated mood (euphoria)</li><li>Agitation and irritability</li><li>Dislike of interference and intolerance of criticism</li><li>Increase in talking and activities</li><li>Flight of ideas – Rapid, continuous speech with sudden and frequent topic change</li><li>Grandiose view of self and abilities (grandiosity)</li><li>Impulsivity – Spending money or giving away money or possessions</li><li>Demanding and manipulative behavior</li><li>Distractibility</li><li>Poor judgment</li><li>Attention-seeking behavior – Flashy dress and makeup or inappropriate behavior</li><li>Impairment in social and occupational functioning</li><li>Decreased sleep</li><li>Neglect of ADLs, including nutrition and hydration</li><li>Possible presence of delusions and hallucinations</li><li>Denial of illness</li></ul>	<ul><li>Flat, blunted or labile affect</li><li>Tearfulness or crying</li><li>Lack of energy</li><li>Anhedonia – Loss of pleasure and lack of interest in activities, hobbies, or sexual activity</li><li>Physical findings of discomfort or pain</li><li>Difficulty concentrating, focusing, and problem solving</li><li>Self-destructive behavior</li><li>Decrease in personal hygiene</li><li>Loss or increase in appetite or sleep, disturbed sleep</li><li>Psychomotor retardation or agitation</li></ul>

- Standardized Screening Tool

    o Mood Disorders Questionnaire

        ▪ The Mood Disorders Questionnaire is a standardized tool that places mood progression on a continuum for hypomania (euphoria) to acute mania (extreme irritability and hyperactivity) to delirium (completely out of touch with reality).

Collaborative Care

- Nursing Care

    o The care of clients with bipolar disorder will be based on the phase of mania clients are experiencing. Nursing care is provided throughout this process.

    o Acute phase

        ▪ Focus is on safety and maintaining physical health.

- Therapeutic milieu (within acute care mental health facility)
  - Provide a safe environment during the acute phase.
  - Evaluate clients regularly for suicidal thoughts, intentions, and escalating behavior.
  - Decrease stimulation without isolating clients if possible. Be aware of noise, music, television, and other clients, all of which may lead to an escalation of the client's behavior. In certain cases, seclusion may be the only way to safely decrease stimulation for this client.
  - Follow agency protocols for providing clients protection (restraints, seclusion, one-to-one observation) if a threat of self-injury or injury to others exists.
  - Implement frequent rest periods.
  - Observe clients closely for escalating behavior.
  - Provide outlets for physical activity. Do not involve clients in activities that last a long time or require a high level of concentration or detailed instructions.
  - Maintenance of self-care needs includes:
    - Monitoring sleep, fluid intake, and nutrition
    - Providing portable, nutritious food because clients may not be able to sit down to eat
    - Supervising choice of clothes
    - Giving step-by-step reminders for hygiene and dress
  - Communication
    - Use a calm, matter-of-fact, specific approach.
    - Give concise explanations.
    - Provide for consistency among staff members.
    - Avoid power struggles, and do not react personally to the client's comments.
    - Listen to and act on legitimate client grievances.
    - Reinforce nonmanipulative behaviors.

(M) **View Media Supplement:** Understanding Bipolar Disorder (Video)

- Medications
  - Mood stabilizers
    - Lithium carbonate (Eskalith)
    - Antiepileptic agents that act as mood stabilizers, including valproic acid (Depakote), clonazepam (Klonopin), lamotrigine (Lamictal), gabapentin (Neurontin), and topiramate (Topamax)
  - Use benzodiazepine (lorazepam [Ativan]) on a short-term basis for a client experiencing sleep impairment related to mania.
  - Use an antidepressant (fluoxetine [Prozac]) to manage a major depressive episode.
  - Use an antipsychotic (risperidone [Risperdal]) to manage psychotic disturbances during the manic phase.
- Therapeutic Procedures
  - Electroconvulsive therapy (ECT) can be useful to subdue extreme manic behavior, especially when pharmacologic therapy, such as lithium, has not worked. ECT can also be used for clients who are suicidal or those with rapid cycling.
  - Nursing Actions
    - A specially trained nurse is responsible for monitoring the client before and after this therapy.
    - Ensure clients have been evaluated for cardiovascular disease, neuromuscular disorders, and complicated pregnancy prior to beginning this treatment.
- Care After Discharge
  - Client Education
  - Management of the continuation and maintenance phases.
    - Recommend case management for follow up of clients and their families.
    - Encourage group, family, and individual psychotherapy to improve problem-solving and interpersonal skills.
    - Reinforce health teaching regarding:
      - The chronicity of the disorder requiring long-term pharmacological and psychological support
      - Indications of impending relapse and ways to manage the crisis
      - Precipitating factors of relapse (sleep disturbance; use of alcohol, caffeine, drugs of abuse)
      - The importance of maintaining a regular sleep, meal, and activity pattern
      - Medication administration and the importance of adherence to the regimen

- Client Outcomes

  - The client will refrain from self-harm.

  - The client will rest 4 to 6 hr per night.

  - The client will maintain adequate fluid and food intake.

  - The client will use appropriate communication skills to meet needs.

  - The client will participate in self-care.

  - The client will not experience relapse.

Complications

- Physical Exhaustion and Possible Death

  - A client in a true manic state usually will not stop moving and does not eat, drink, or sleep. These episodes can last for weeks or months depending on how long the client is in the manic state. The longer the client is in the manic state, the greater the risks for psychotic episodes. This can become a medical emergency.

  - Nursing Actions

    - Prevent client self-harm.

    - Decrease client's physical activity.

    - Promote adequate fluid and food intake.

    - Ensure a minimum of 4 to 6 hr of sleep each night.

    - Assist the client with self-care needs.

    - Manage medication appropriately.

(A) APPLICATION EXERCISES

Scenario: A client in the manic phase of bipolar I disorder is being admitted to an inpatient acute care mental health unit. The provider's plan is for this client to undergo electroconvulsive therapy (ECT) during the first week of hospitalization. The client has been admitted several times in the past, and his behavior has typically caused upheaval in the unit. The staff is talking negatively about the client even before the client's arrival.

1. List the communication principles the nurse manager on the unit should review with the staff regarding this client.

2. After 1 week on the acute care mental health unit, the client's mania has decreased somewhat. However, the client has periodic episodes of irritability. What nursing interventions could help reduce the client's irritability?

3. A client who has bipolar I disorder is in the acute phase and unable to eat or sleep. The client's moods change rapidly from elated to agitated. If this client threatens to hit a staff member or another client, which of the following verbal responses by the nurse is appropriate?

   A. "You will be put in seclusion and kept there if you make any more threats."

   B. "Do not hit him or me. If you cannot control yourself, we will help you."

   C. "That's enough! You know we do not tolerate this type of behavior."

   D. "That will only make things worse. Why would you want to hurt someone?"

4. A client who has bipolar I disorder is standing with a group of clients in the mental health unit. The client is talking excitedly and at great length about a variety of topics. The nurse can see that the other clients are becoming anxious and restless but do not know what to do to stop the conversation. Which of the following is the first action the nurse should take?

   A. Give honest feedback.

   B. Administer a sedative.

   C. Set limits.

   D. Use distraction.

APPLICATION EXERCISES ANSWER KEY

Scenario: A client in the manic phase of bipolar I disorder is being admitted to an inpatient acute care mental health unit. The provider's plan is for this client to undergo electroconvulsive therapy (ECT) during the first week of hospitalization. The client has been admitted several times in the past, and his behavior has typically caused upheaval in the unit. The staff is talking negatively about the client even before the client's arrival.

1. List the communication principles the nurse manager on the unit should review with the staff regarding this client.

    Use a firm, calm approach.

    Give explanations in a short, concise manner.

    Refrain from responding personally to the client's comments.

    Be consistent in approach and expectations.

    Talk with other staff members about which techniques work and which do not.

    Adhere to agreed-upon limits.

    Let the client know the consequences of inappropriate behavior.

    Hear and act on legitimate complaints.

     NCLEX® Connection: Psychosocial Integrity, Therapeutic Communications

2. After 1 week on the acute care mental health unit, the client's mania has decreased somewhat. However, the client has periodic episodes of irritability. What nursing interventions could help reduce the client's irritability?

    Use a calm, matter-of-fact, specific approach.

    Reduce environmental stimulation.

    Implement frequent rest periods.

    Provide outlets for physical activity.

     NCLEX® Connection: Psychosocial Integrity, Therapeutic Environment

3. A client who has bipolar I disorder is in the acute phase and unable to eat or sleep. The client's moods change rapidly from elated to agitated. If this client threatens to hit a staff member or another client, which of the following verbal responses by the nurse is appropriate?

    A. "You will be put in seclusion and kept there if you make any more threats."

    B. "Do not hit him or me. If you cannot control yourself, we will help you."

    C. "That's enough! You know we do not tolerate this type of behavior."

    D. "That will only make things worse. Why would you want to hurt someone?"

    The correct response is to set limits in concrete, simple sentences to de-escalate the situation. Option A threatens the client with seclusion as a punishment and is assault. Option C does not help the client stop her behavior. Option D asks a question the client cannot answer.

    (N) NCLEX® Connection: Psychosocial Integrity, Therapeutic Communications

4. A client who has bipolar I disorder is standing with a group of clients in the mental health unit. The client is talking excitedly and at great length about a variety of topics. The nurse can see that the other clients are becoming anxious and restless but do not know what to do to stop the conversation. Which of the following is the first action the nurse should take?

    A. Give honest feedback.

    B. Administer a sedative.

    C. Set limits.

    D. Use distraction.

    The client is most likely in the acute phase and can easily be distracted. The nurse should first try using distraction because it is the least invasive intervention. Giving feedback, administering a sedative, and setting limits are all appropriate actions but not the least invasive.

    (N) NCLEX® Connection: Psychosocial Integrity, Behavioral Interventions

UNIT 3	PSYCHOBIOLOGIC DISORDERS
Chapter 13	Schizophrenia

Overview

- Schizophrenia is a group of psychotic disorders that affect thinking, behavior, emotions, and the ability to perceive reality.

- Schizophrenia may result from a combination of genetic and nongenetic factors (injury at birth, nutritional factors, viral infection, hormonal imbalances).

- The typical age of onset is late teens and early 20s, but schizophrenia has occurred in young children and may begin in later adulthood.

- A diagnosis of schizophrenia should not be made for children until after age 7 to rule out attention deficit hyperactivity disorder (ADHD) with violent tendencies.

- Schizophrenia becomes problematic when clinical manifestations interfere with interpersonal relationships, self-care, and ability to work.

- Categories and Taxonomies of Disorder

  o The various types of schizophrenia recognized and defined by the DSM-IV-TR include:

TYPE OF SCHIZOPHRENIA	COMMON SYMPTOMS
Paranoid - Characterized by suspicion toward others	- Hallucinations (hearing threatening voices) and delusions (believing oneself President of the United States) - Other-directed violence may occur.
Disorganized - Characterized by withdrawal from society and very inappropriate behaviors (poor hygiene, muttering constantly to oneself) - Frequently seen in the homeless population	- Loose associations - Bizarre mannerisms - Incoherent speech - Hallucinations and delusions may be present but are much less organized than those seen in clients with paranoia.

TYPE OF SCHIZOPHRENIA	COMMON SYMPTOMS

Catatonic
• Characterized by abnormal motor movements
• Stages
   ○ Withdrawn
   ○ Excited
	Withdrawn stage
	• Psychomotor retardation – Clients may appear comatose.
	• Waxy flexibility may be present.
	• Clients often have extreme self-care needs (tube feeding due to an inability to eat).
	Excited stage
	• Constant movement, unusual posturing, and incoherent speech
	• Self-care needs may predominate.
	• Clients may be a danger to self or others.

Residual • Active clinical manifestations are no longer present, but clients have two or more "residual" findings.	• Anergia, anhedonia, or avolition • Withdrawal from social activities • Impaired role function • Speech problems (alogia) • Odd behaviors (walking in a strange way)
Undifferentiated • Clients have clinical manifestations of schizophrenia but do not meet criteria for any of the other types.	• Any positive or negative symptoms may be present.

- Other psychotic disorders include:

    - Schizoaffective disorder – The client's disorder meets both the criteria for schizophrenia and one of the affective disorders (depression, mania, a mixed disorder).

        - Often the client is in the acute phase of bipolar I disorder with characteristics of psychosis.

    - Brief psychotic disorder – Clients have psychotic clinical manifestations that last between 1 day to 1 month in duration.

    - Schizophreniform disorder – Clients have clinical manifestations like those of schizophrenia, but the duration is from 1 to 6 months and social/occupational dysfunction may or may not be present.

        - Often the provider will diagnose clients with schizophreniform until further evaluation can be made to decide if the client has schizophrenia or schizoaffective disorder

    - Shared psychotic disorder – One person begins to share the delusional beliefs of another person with psychosis. This is also called folie à deux.

    - Secondary (induced) psychosis – Signs of psychosis are brought on by a medical disorder (Alzheimer's disease) or by use of chemical substances (alcohol abuse).

Data Collection

- Subjective and Objective Data

CHARACTERISTIC DIMENSIONS OF SCHIZOPHRENIA	
CHARACTERISTICS	EXAMPLES OF BEHAVIOR IN EACH DIMENSION
Positive symptoms • These are the most easily identified clinical manifestations.	• Hallucinations • Delusions • Alterations in speech • Bizarre behavior (walking backward constantly)
Negative symptoms • These clinical manifestations are more difficult to treat successfully than positive symptoms.	• Affect – Usually blunted (narrow range of normal expression) or flat (facial expression never changes) • Alogia – Poverty of thought or speech. Clients may sit with a visitor but may only mumble or respond vaguely to questions. • Avolition – Lack of motivation in activities and hygiene. Clients complete an assigned task (making the bed) but are unable to start the next common chore without prompting. • Anhedonia – Lack of pleasure or joy. Clients are indifferent to things that often make others happy (looking at beautiful scenery). • Anergia – Lack of energy

Cognitive symptoms
• Problems with thinking make it very difficult for clients to live independently.
	• Disordered thinking
	• Inability to make decisions
	• Poor problem-solving ability
	• Difficulty concentrating to perform tasks
	• Memory deficits
	  ○ Long-term memory
	  ○ Working memory (inability to follow directions to find an address)

Depressive symptoms	• Hopelessness • Suicidal ideation

○ Alterations in thought (delusions) are false fixed beliefs that cannot be corrected by reasoning and are usually bizarre. These include:

DELUSIONS	EXAMPLES
Ideas of reference	Misconstrue trivial events and attach personal significance to them (believing that others, who are discussing the next meal, are talking about them)
Persecution	Feel singled out for harm by others (being hunted down by the FBI)
Grandeur	Believe that they are all powerful and important, like a god
Somatic delusions	Believe that their body is changing in an unusual way (growing a third arm)
Jealousy	May feel that their spouse is sexually involved with another individual
Being controlled	Believe that a force outside their body controls them
Thought broadcasting	Believes that their thoughts are heard by others
Thought insertion	Believe that others' thoughts are being inserted into their mind
Thought withdrawal	Believes that their thoughts have been removed from their mind by an outside agency
Religiosity	Is obsessed with religious beliefs

○ The following are examples of alterations in speech that can occur with schizophrenia:

ALTERATIONS IN SPEECH	
Flight of ideas	• Associative looseness • Clients may say sentence after sentence, but each sentence may relate to another topic, and the listener is unable to follow the client's thoughts.
Neologisms	• Made up words that only have meaning to the client, such as, "I tranged and flittled."
Echolalia	• Clients repeat the words spoken to them.
Clang association	• Meaningless rhyming of words, often forceful, such as, "Oh fox, box, and lox."
Word salad	• Words jumbled together with little meaning or significance to listener, such as, "Hip hooray, the flip is cast and wide-sprinting in the forest."

○ Alterations in perception

■ Hallucinations are sensory perceptions that do not have any apparent external stimulus. Examples include:

□ Auditory – Hearing voices or sounds that may take the form of commands instructing clients to hurt self or others

□ Visual – Seeing people or things

□ Olfactory – Smelling odors

□ Gustatory – Experiencing tastes

□ Tactile – Feeling bodily sensations

- Personal boundary difficulties – Disenfranchisement with one's own body, identity, and perceptions. This includes:
  □ Depersonalization – Nonspecific feeling that a person has lost her identity; self is different or unreal
  □ Derealization – Perception that environment has changed
- Alterations in behavior
  □ Extreme agitation, including pacing and rocking
  □ Stereotyped behaviors – Motor patterns that had meaning to the client (sweeping the floor) but now are mechanical and lack purpose
  □ Automatic obedience – Responding in a robot-like manner
  □ Wavy flexibility – Excessive maintenance of position
  □ Stupor – Motionless for long periods of time (coma-like)
  □ Negativism – Doing the opposite of what is requested
  □ Echopraxia – Purposeful imitation of movements made by others
- Standardized Screening Tools
  ○ The Global Assessment of Functioning (GAF) scale – Helps to determine a client's ability to perform ADLs and to function independently
  ○ Scale for Assessment of Negative Symptoms
  ○ Simpson Neurological Rating Scale

Collaborative Care

- Nursing Care
  ○ Use milieu therapy for clients who have schizophrenia both in 24-hr mental health facilities and in community facilities, such as adult day care programs.
    - Provide a structured, safe environment (milieu) for clients in order to decrease anxiety and to distract them from constant thinking about hallucinations.
  ○ Promote therapeutic communication to lower anxiety, decrease defensive patterns, and encourage participation in the milieu.
  ○ Establish a trusting relationship with clients.
  ○ Encourage the development of social skills and friendships.
  ○ Encourage participation in group work and psychotherapy.
  ○ Use appropriate communication to address hallucinations and delusions.
    - Ask clients directly about hallucinations. The nurse should not argue or agree with client's view of the situation, but may offer a comment, such as, "I don't hear anything, but you seem to be feeling frightened."

- Do not argue with a client's delusions, but focus on the client's feelings and possibly offer reasonable explanations, such as, "I can't imagine that the President of the United States would have a reason to kill a citizen, but it must be frightening for you to believe that."

- Provide for safety if clients are experiencing command hallucinations.

- Attempt to focus conversations on reality-based subjects.

- Identify symptom triggers, such as loud noises (may trigger auditory hallucinations in certain clients), and situations that seem to trigger conversations about the client's delusions.

- Be genuine and empathetic in all dealings with clients.

o Determine discharge needs, such as ability to perform ADLs.

o Promote self-care by modeling and instructing clients about self-care activities within the mental health facility.

o Relate wellness to the elements of symptom management.

o Collaborate with clients in the use of symptom management techniques to cope with depressive clinical manifestations and anxiety. Symptom management techniques include such strategies as using music to distract from "voices," attending activities, walking, talking to a trusted person when hallucinations are most bothersome, and interacting with an auditory or visual hallucination by telling it to stop or go away.

o Encourage medication compliance.

o Reinforce teaching regarding medications.

USE OF MEDICATIONS	EXAMPLES OF MEDICATION	TEACHING
Atypical antipsychotics are current medications of choice for psychotic disorders, and they generally treat both positive and negative symptoms.	• Risperidone (Risperdal) • Olanzapine (Zyprexa) • Quetiapine (Seroquel) • Ziprasidone (Geodon) • Aripiprazole (Abilify) • Clozapine (Clozaril)	• To minimize weight gain, advise clients to follow a healthy, low-calorie diet, engage in regular exercise, and monitor weight gain. • Clinical manifestations of agitation, dizziness, sedation, and sleep disruption may occur. Instruct clients to report these side effects to his provider, as the medication may need to be changed.
Conventional antipsychotics are used to treat mainly positive psychotic symptoms.	• Haloperidol (Haldol) • Loxapine (Loxitane) • Chlorpromazine (Thorazine) • Fluphenazine (Prolixin)	• To minimize anticholinergic effects, advise clients to chew sugarless gum, eat foods high in fiber, and eat and drink 2 to 3 L of fluid per day. • Instruct clients about clinical findings of postural hypotension (light-headedness, dizziness). If these occur, advise clients to sit or lie down. Orthostatic hypotension can be minimized by getting up slowly from a lying or sitting position. • Monitor clients for extrapyramidal side effects.

USE OF MEDICATIONS	EXAMPLES OF MEDICATION	TEACHING
Antidepressants are used to treat the depression seen in many clients with schizophrenia.	• Paroxetine (Paxil)	• Used temporarily to treat depression associated with schizophrenia. • Monitor clients for suicidal ideation, as this medication may increase thoughts of self-harm, especially when first taking it. • Notify the provider of any side effects, such as deepened depression. • Advise clients to avoid abrupt cessation of this medication to avoid a withdrawal effect.
Anxiolytics/ benzodiazepines are used to treat the anxiety often found in clients with schizophrenia, as well as some of the positive and negative symptoms of schizophrenia.	• Lorazepam (Ativan) • Clonazepam (Klonopin)	• Inform clients of this medication's sedative effects. • Inform clients the need for blood tests to monitor for agranulocytosis. • These medications are used with caution in older adult clients.

(M) View Media Supplement: Understanding Schizophrenia (Video)

- Care After Discharge

    o Client Education

        ▪ Recommend case management to provide for follow up of clients and their families.

        ▪ Encourage group, family, and individual psychotherapy to improve problem-solving and interpersonal skills

        ▪ Reinforce teaching regarding the following:

            □ Need for self-care to prevent relapse

            □ Medication effects, side effects, and importance of adherence to the regimen

            □ Importance of attending support groups

            □ Abstinence from the use of alcohol and/or drugs

            □ Keeping a log or journal of feelings and changes in behavior to help monitor medication effectiveness

- Client Outcomes

    o The client will regularly attend support groups.

    o The client will maintain an appropriate level of self-care.

    o The client will maintain medication adherence.

(A) APPLICATION EXERCISES

1. A 19-year-old college student comes to a mental health emergency facility experiencing hallucinations. Which strategies should the nurse at the facility use when working with this client?

2. Positive symptoms of schizophrenia include which of the following? (Select all that apply.)

   _____ Auditory hallucinations

   _____ Lack of motivation

   _____ Minimal to no energy

   _____ Delusions of persecution

   _____ Motor agitation

   _____ Flat affect

3. A client who has schizophrenia has great difficulty with personal boundaries. Which of the following is a personal boundary problem?

   A. Delusions of grandeur

   B. Depersonalization

   C. Visual hallucinations

   D. Poverty of speech

4. Match the symptoms below with the appropriate psychotic disorders.

   _____ Schizophreniform disorder   A. Psychotic symptoms caused by abuse of chemical substances or physical illness

   _____ Schizoaffective disorder   B. An absence of active symptoms of schizophrenia with two or more persistent or lingering symptoms

   _____ Shared psychotic disorder   C. Psychotic behavior lasting between 1 and 6 months that may not impair the client's ability to function at work or in social situations

   _____ Residual schizophrenia   D. Symptoms of schizophrenia along with symptoms of mania or major depression

   _____ Induced psychosis   E. One person sharing the delusional beliefs of a person who has psychosis

5. A nurse is caring for a client on an inpatient mental health unit. The client says to the nurse, "I want a bomin with a chockle on top for my hapsoma." This is an example of which of the following speech alterations?

   A. Word salad

   B. Neologisms

   C. Clang associations

   D. Echolalia

APPLICATION EXERCISES ANSWER KEY

1. A 19-year-old college student comes to a mental health emergency facility experiencing hallucinations. Which strategies should the nurse at the facility use when working with this client?

   Establish a trusting nurse-client relationship.

   Observe the characteristics of the hallucinations, including duration, intensity, frequency, and type.

   Focus on the symptom – the "feelings" – and ask the client to describe what is happening.

   Determine whether or not the client has used drugs or alcohol.

   If asked, point out that you are not experiencing the same stimuli.

   Help the client describe and compare current and past hallucinations.

   Assist the client in identifying needs that may be reflected in the content of the hallucinations.

   Determine the impact of the client's symptoms on ADLs.

   NCLEX® Connection: Psychosocial Integrity, Mental Health Concepts

2. Positive symptoms of schizophrenia include which of the following? (Select all that apply.)

__X__	**Auditory hallucinations**
_____	Lack of motivation
_____	Minimal to no energy
__X__	**Delusions of persecution**
__X__	**Motor agitation**
_____	Flat affect

   Auditory hallucinations, delusions of persecution, and motor agitation are all positive symptoms of schizophrenia. Lack of motivation (avolition), minimal to no energy (anergia), and flat affect (facial expression) are negative symptoms.

   NCLEX® Connection: Physiological Adaptations, Basic Pathophysiology

3. A client who has schizophrenia has great difficulty with personal boundaries. Which of the following is a personal boundary problem?

   A. Delusions of grandeur

   B. Depersonalization

   C. Visual hallucinations

   D. Poverty of speech

   Depersonalization (a feeling of being separated from one's body) is an example of a problem with personal boundaries. Delusions and hallucinations are positive symptoms of schizophrenia. Poverty of speech or thought (alogia) is a negative symptom of schizophrenia.

   Ⓝ NCLEX® Connection: Psychosocial Integrity, Mental Health Concepts

4. Match the symptoms below with the appropriate psychotic disorders.

__C__	Schizophreniform disorder	A. Psychotic symptoms caused by abuse of chemical substances or physical illness
__D__	Schizoaffective disorder	B. An absence of active symptoms of schizophrenia with two or more persistent or lingering symptoms
__E__	Shared psychotic disorder	C. Psychotic behavior lasting between 1 and 6 months that may not impair the client's ability to function at work or in social situations
__B__	Residual schizophrenia	D. Symptoms of schizophrenia along with symptoms of mania or major depression
__A__	Induced psychosis	E. One person sharing the delusional beliefs of a person who has psychosis

   Ⓝ NCLEX® Connection: Physiological Adaptations, Basic Pathophysiology

5. A nurse is caring for a client on an inpatient mental health unit. The client says to the nurse, "I want a bomin with a chockle on top for my hapsoma." This is an example of which of the following speech alterations?

   A. Word salad

   B. Neologisms

   C. Clang associations

   D. Echolalia

   Neologisms are fabricated words that only have meaning to the client. Word salad is a jumble of actual words that have little meaning or significance to the listener. Clang associations are meaningless rhymes of words. Echolalia is a repetition of words the client hears.

   Ⓝ NCLEX® Connection: Psychosocial Integrity, Mental Health Concepts

UNIT 3	PSYCHOBIOLOGIC DISORDERS
Chapter 14	Personality Disorders

Overview

- Clients who have personality disorders demonstrate long-term maladaptive behavior that prevents accomplishment of desired goals in relationships and other efforts.

- The maladaptive behaviors of a personality disorder are not experienced as uncomfortable by the individual, and some areas of personal functioning may be very adequate.

- Personality disorders are predisposing factors for many other psychiatric disorders and often co-occur with depression and anxiety.

- Personality disorders have a significant effect on the course of treatment for other psychiatric disorders.

- The various personality disorders recognized and defined by the DSM-IV-TR are as follows:

  o Cluster A – Generally described as odd or eccentric

  o Cluster B – Generally described as dramatic, emotional, or erratic

  o Cluster C – Generally described as anxious or fearful

- Defense mechanisms used by clients who have personality disorders include repression, suppression, regression, undoing, and splitting.

  o Of these, splitting, which is the inability to incorporate positive and negative aspects of oneself or others into a whole image, is frequently seen in the inpatient setting.

  o Splitting is commonly associated with borderline personality disorder.

  o In splitting, clients tend to characterize people or things as all good or all bad at any particular moment. For example, the client might say, "You are the worst person in the world." Later that day she might say, "You are the best, but the nurse from the last shift is absolutely terrible."

Data Collection

- Risk Factors

  o Individuals who have personality disorders tend to be less educated or unemployed, are single or have marital difficulties, often have comorbid substance use disorders, and may commit nonviolent and violent crimes, including sex offenses.

- Environmental influences (child abuse), biological influences (genetic factors), and psychological factors, appear to play a role in the etiology of personality disorders.
- Subjective and Objective Data
  - All personality disorders share four common characteristics:
    - Inflexibility/maladaptive responses to stress
    - Disability in social and professional relationships
    - Tendency to provoke interpersonal conflict
    - Ability to merge personal boundaries with others

THE 10 PERSONALITY DISORDERS	
Cluster A (odd or eccentric traits)	
Paranoid	• Characterized by distrust and suspiciousness toward others based on unfounded beliefs that others want to harm, exploit, or deceive the person
Schizoid	• Characterized by emotional detachment, disinterest in close relationships, and indifference to praise or criticism • Often uncooperative • Differs from schizophrenia in that clients do not have psychotic symptoms
Schizotypal	• Characterized by odd beliefs leading to interpersonal difficulties, an eccentric appearance, and magical thinking or perceptual distortions that are not clear delusions or hallucinations
Cluster B (dramatic, emotional, or erratic traits)	
Antisocial	• Characterized by disregard for others with exploitation, repeated unlawful actions, deceit, and failure to accept personal responsibility
Borderline	• Characterized by instability of affect, identity, and relationships • Fear of abandonment, splitting behaviors, manipulation, and impulsiveness • Often tries self-mutilation and may be suicidal
Histrionic	• Characterized by emotional attention-seeking behavior, in which the person needs to be the center of attention • Often seductive and flirtatious
Narcissistic	• Characterized by arrogance, grandiose views of self-importance, the need for consistent admiration, and a lack of empathy for others that strains most relationships • Often sensitive to criticism • May have clinical manifestations of grandiosity

THE 10 PERSONALITY DISORDERS	
Cluster C (anxious or fearful traits; insecurity and inadequacy)	
Avoidant	• Characterized by social inhibition and avoidance of all situations that require interpersonal contact, despite wanting close relationships, due to extreme fear of rejection • Often very anxious in social situations • Afraid of being criticized or ridiculed and will avoid situations where clients believe this might occur
Dependent	• Characterized by extreme dependency in a close relationship with an urgent search to find a replacement when one relationship ends • The most frequently seen personality disorder in the clinical setting • May have somatization symptoms
Obsessive compulsive	• Characterized by perfectionism with a focus on orderliness and control to the extent that the individual may not be able to accomplish a given task • Differs from obsessive compulsive disorder in that clients do not have the need to repeat things in a ritual manner until the they get the right feeling

Collaborative Care

- Nursing Care

  o Perform self-assessment regarding possible feelings of frustration, anger, or fear when caring for clients who have personality disorders. Clients who have personality disorders may evoke intense feelings.

  o Use milieu therapy in a group context aimed at the specific personality disorder.

  o Provide for safety because some clients who have a personality disorder are at risk for self- or other-directed violence.

  o Communication strategies

    ■ Developing a therapeutic relationship is often challenging because of the client's distrust or hostility toward others. Feelings of being threatened or having no control may cause a client to act out toward a nurse.

      □ Use a firm, yet supportive approach and consistent care to help build a therapeutic nurse-client relationship.

      □ Offer clients realistic choices to enhance the their sense of control.

      □ Use limit-setting and consistency with clients who are manipulative, especially those with borderline or antisocial personality disorders.

      □ Encourage assertiveness training and modeling for clients who have dependent and histrionic personality disorders.

      □ Model behavior for Clients who have personality disorders.

      □ Maintain professional boundaries and communication with clients who have a histrionic personality disorder, who may be very flirtatious.

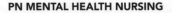

- ☐ Respect the need for social isolation for clients who have schizoid or schizotypal personality disorder.

- ☐ Self-assess frequently for countertransference reactions to very dependent clients who are clingy and frequently requesting help.

- Medications

  - ○ Use psychotropic agents that are geared toward maintaining cognitive function and relieving symptoms. Other medications used include antidepressants, anxiolytics, or a combination of these medications.

- Interdisciplinary Care

  - ○ Psychobiological interventions include the following:

    - ■ Use dialectical behavior therapy, a cognitive-behavioral therapy, for clients who have borderline personality disorder. It focuses on gradual behavior changes and provides acceptance and validation for these clients, who are very frequently (80% of cases) suicidal and have self-mutilating behaviors.

    - ■ Use case management for clients who have personality disorders and are persistently and severely impaired.

      - ☐ In acute care facilities, case management focuses on obtaining pertinent history from current or previous providers, supporting reintegration with the family, and ensuring appropriate referrals to outpatient care.

      - ☐ In long-term outpatient facilities, case management goals include reducing hospitalization by providing resources for crisis services and enhancing the social support system.

- Client Outcomes

  - ○ The client will identify methods for problem solving.

  - ○ The client will remain free from harm.

  - ○ The client will assume responsibility for own actions.

  - ○ The client will demonstrate the ability to function in society.

Ⓐ APPLICATION EXERCISES

1. A nurse on an inpatient psychiatric unit is asked to conduct a staff in-service program about communicating with clients who have personality disorders. The nursing staff includes RNs, LPNs, and mental health technicians. Although some of them have previous mental health work experience, no one has worked in a mental health facility for more than 5 years, and there is disagreement among the staff about the best strategies for dealing with clients who have personality disorders. Identify three components of care that are important to include in the in-service.

2. Match the letter of the description with the personality disorder to which it corresponds.

_____	Borderline	A.	Perfectionistic and orderly; demands control of every situation
_____	Narcissistic	B.	Evades all social situations and fears rejection
_____	Obsessive-compulsive	C.	Emotionally detached, uncooperative, and disinterested in others
_____	Dependent	D.	Arrogant, with grandiose views of self-importance and a need for admiration
_____	Avoidant	E.	Emotional with unstable identity and relationships; fears abandonment
_____	Schizoid	F.	Excessively reliant on others in a close relationship

3. When a client who has borderline personality disorder asks his roommate to play a card game with him and the roommate agrees, the client says, "You are my very best friend in this place." Later the client asks the roommate if he can borrow his magazine and the roommate says not until after he finishes reading it himself. The client says, "I hate you. You are so evil for not sharing." This is an example of

   A. regression.
   B. splitting.
   C. undoing.
   D. identification.

4. A client who has antisocial personality disorder is admitted to a chemical dependency unit. The nurse should be alert for which of the following characteristic behaviors of clients with this type of personality disorder? (Select all that apply.)

   _____ Submissive
   _____ Indecisive
   _____ Exploitative
   _____ Irresponsible
   _____ Deceptive
   _____ Unlawful

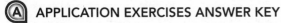

APPLICATION EXERCISES ANSWER KEY

1. A nurse on an inpatient psychiatric unit is asked to conduct a staff in-service program about communicating with clients who have personality disorders. The nursing staff includes RNs, LPNs, and mental health technicians. Although some of them have previous mental health work experience, no one has worked in a mental health facility for more than 5 years, and there is disagreement among the staff about the best strategies for dealing with clients who have personality disorders. Identify three components of care that are important to include in the in-service.

   Clients who have personality disorders have a tendency to cause frustration and stress in those caring for them. Self-awareness is important when providing care for these clients in order to maintain professionalism and enhance the client's well-being. Effective communication among staff is also important, as many clients who have personality disorders use various defense mechanisms in an effort to get their needs met. Limit-setting is often necessary with clients who have personality disorders. Other important topics to cover are establishing trust with these clients (who are likely to be mistrustful of health care professionals), keeping them safe, and enhancing their involvement in and sense of control over their care.

   NCLEX® Connection: Psychosocial Integrity, Behavioral Interventions

2. Match the letter of the description with the personality disorder to which it corresponds.

E	Borderline	A. Perfectionistic and orderly; demands control of every situation
D	Narcissistic	B. Evades all social situations and fears rejection
A	Obsessive-compulsive	C. Emotionally detached, uncooperative, and disinterested in others
F	Dependent	D. Arrogant, with grandiose views of self-importance and a need for admiration
B	Avoidant	E. Emotional with unstable identity and relationships; fears abandonment
C	Schizoid	F. Excessively reliant on others in a close relationship

   NCLEX® Connection: Psychosocial Integrity, Mental Health Concepts

3. When a client who has borderline personality disorder asks his roommate to play a card game with him and the roommate agrees, the client says, "You are my very best friend in this place." Later the client asks the roommate if he can borrow his magazine and the roommate says not until after he finishes reading it himself. The client says, "I hate you. You are so evil for not sharing." This is an example of

   A. regression.

   B. splitting.

   C. undoing.

   D. identification.

   Splitting occurs when a person is unable to see both positive and negative qualities at the same time. Clients who have borderline personality disorders tend to see a person as all bad one time and all good another time. Regression refers to resorting to an earlier way of functioning, such as having a temper tantrum. Undoing is an attempt to make up for a previous action or altercation. With identification, clients imitate the behavior of someone they admire or fear.

   Ⓝ NCLEX® Connection: Psychosocial Integrity, Mental Health Concepts

4. A client who has antisocial personality disorder is admitted to a chemical dependency unit. The nurse should be alert for which of the following characteristic behaviors of clients with this type of personality disorder? (Select all that apply.)

_____	Submissive
_____	Indecisive
__X__	**Exploitative**
__X__	**Irresponsible**
__X__	**Deceptive**
__X__	**Unlawful**

   Clients who have antisocial personality disorders typically display behavior that is exploitative, irresponsible, deceptive, and unlawful. They rarely appear submissive or indecisive.

   Ⓝ NCLEX® Connection: Psychosocial Integrity, Mental Health Concepts

UNIT 3	PSYCHOBIOLOGIC DISORDERS
Chapter 15	Cognitive Disorders

◎ Overview

- Cognitive disorders are a group of conditions characterized by the disruption of thinking, memory, processing, and problem solving.

- Treatment of clients with cognitive disorders requires a compassionate understanding of both clients and their families.

- The various cognitive disorders recognized and defined by the DSM-IV-TR include:

  o Delirium

  o Dementia

  o Amnestic disorders

Data Collection

- Risk Factors

  o Risk factors for cognitive disorders include physiological changes, such as neurological (Parkinson's disease, Huntington's disease), metabolic (hepatic or renal failure, fluid and electrolyte imbalances, nutritional deficiencies), and cardiovascular diseases; family genetics; infections (HIV/AIDS); tumors; substance abuse; drug intoxication; and drug withdrawal.

  o Risk factors for Alzheimer's disease include advanced age, female gender, prior head trauma, and a family history of Alzheimer's disease or trisomy (Down syndrome).

- Subjective and Objective Data

  o Delirium and dementia have some similarities and some important differences:

DELIRIUM	DEMENTIA
Onset	
• Rapid over a short period of time (hours or days)	• Gradual deterioration of function over months or years
Clinical Manifestations	
• Occurrence of impairments in memory, judgment, ability to focus, and ability to calculate. These impairments may fluctuate throughout the day. • Level of consciousness is usually altered. • Restlessness and agitation are common. Sundowning (confusion during the night) may occur. Behaviors may increase or decrease daily. • Personality change is rapid. • Some perceptual disturbances may be present (hallucinations and illusions). • Vital signs may be unstable and abnormal due to medical illness.	• Impairments in memory, judgment, speech (aphasia), ability to recognize familiar objects (agnosia), executive functioning (managing daily tasks), and movement (apraxia). Impairments do not change throughout the day. • Level of consciousness is usually unchanged. • Restlessness and agitation are common. Sundowning may occur. Behaviors usually remain stable. • Personality change is gradual. • Vital signs are stable unless other illness is present.
Cause	
• Caused secondary to another medical condition, such as infection (in older adults), or to substance abuse	• Generally caused by a chronic disease (Alzheimer's disease) or is the result of chronic alcohol abuse • May be caused by permanent trauma (head injury)
Outcome	
• Reversible if diagnosis and treatment are prompt	• Irreversible and progressive

STAGES OF ALZHEIMER'S DISEASE	
STAGE	**CLINICAL MANIFESTATIONS**
Stage 1: No impairment (normal function)	• No memory problems • No memory problems evident to provider
Stage 2: Very mild cognitive decline, which may be normal age-related changes, or very early signs of Alzheimer's disease	• Forgetfulness, especially of everyday objects (eyeglasses, wallet) • No memory problems evident to provider, friends, or coworkers

STAGES OF ALZHEIMER'S DISEASE	
STAGE	CLINICAL MANIFESTATIONS
Stage 3: Mild cognitive decline, including problems with memory or concentration that may be measurable in clinical testing or during a detailed medical interview	• Mild cognitive deficits, including losing or misplacing important objects and decreased ability to plan • Short-term memory loss noticeable to close relations • Decreased attention span • Difficulty remembering words or names • Difficulty in social or work situations
Stage 4: Moderate cognitive decline (mild or early-stage Alzheimer's disease) that is clearly detected during a medical interview	• Personality change – Appearing withdrawn or subdued, especially in social or mentally challenging situations • Obvious memory loss • Limited knowledge and memory of recent occasions, current events, or personal history • Difficulty performing tasks that require planning and organizing (paying bills, managing money) • Difficulty with complex mental arithmetic
Stage 5: Moderately severe cognitive decline (moderate or mid-stage Alzheimer's disease)	• Increasing cognitive deficits • Inability to recall important details (address, telephone number), but ability to remember information about self and family • Disorientation and confusion as to time and place
Stage 6: Severe cognitive decline (moderately severe or mid-stage Alzheimer's disease)	• Continued worsening of memory difficulties • Loss of awareness of recent events and surroundings • Ability to recall own name but not personal history • Evidence of significant personality changes (delusions, hallucinations, compulsive behaviors) • Wandering behavior • Assistance required for usual daily activities (dressing, toileting, other grooming) • Disruption of normal sleep/wake cycle • Increased episodes of urinary and fecal incontinence • Violent tendencies with potential danger to self or others
Stage 7: Very severe cognitive decline (severe or late-stage Alzheimer's disease)	• Loss of ability to respond to environment, to speak, and to control movement • Unrecognizable speech, general urinary incontinence, inability to eat without assistance, and impaired swallowing • Gradual loss of all ability to move • Stupor and coma • Death frequently related to choking or infection

- Defense Mechanisms Used in Cognitive Disorders

  o Clients use defense mechanisms to preserve self-esteem when cognitive changes are progressive:

    ▪ Denial – Both clients and family members may refuse to believe that changes, such as loss of memory, are taking place, even when those changes are obvious to others.

    ▪ Confabulation – Clients may make up stories when questioned about events or activities that they do not remember. This may seem like lying, but it is actually an unconscious attempt to save self-esteem and prevent admitting that they do not remember the occasion.

    ▪ Perseveration – Clients avoid answering questions by repeating phrases or behavior. This is another unconscious attempt to maintain self-esteem when memory has failed.

- Amnestic disorder may be secondary to substance abuse or another medical condition. Typically there is no personality change or impairment in abstract thinking. Changes due to amnestic disorder include the following:

  o Decreased awareness of surroundings

  o Inability to learn new information despite normal attention

  o Inability to recall previously learned information

  o Possible disorientation to place and time

- Laboratory and Diagnostic Tests

  o Chest and skull x-rays

  o Electroencephalography (EEG)

  o Electrocardiography (ECG)

  o Liver function studies

  o Thyroid function tests

  o Neuroimaging (computer tomography and position emission tomography of the brain)

  o Urinalysis

  o Serum electrolytes

- Standardized Screening Tools

  o Mini-Mental State Examination (MMSE)

  o Functional Dementia Scale

    ▪ Use of this tool will give the nurse information regarding the client's ability to perform self-care, the extent of the client's memory loss, mood changes, and the degree of danger to self or others.

- o Mini-Mental Status Examination
- o Functional Assessment Screening Tool
- o Global Deterioration Scale
- o Geriatric Depression Scale (short form)
- o Michigan Alcoholism Screening Test – Geriatric Version

Collaborative Care

- Nursing Care
  - o Perform self-assessment regarding possible feelings of frustration, anger, or fear when performing daily care for clients who have progressive dementia.
  - o Nursing interventions are focused on protecting clients from injury, as well as promoting their dignity and quality of life.
  - o Provide a safe and therapeutic environment.
    - Assign clients to a room close to the nurse's station for close observation.
    - Provide a room with a low level of visual and auditory stimuli.
    - Provide for a well-lit environment, minimizing contrasts and shadows.
    - Have clients sit in a room with windows to help with time orientation.
    - Have clients wear an identification bracelet. Use monitors and bed alarm devices as needed.
    - Use restraints only as an intervention of last resort.
    - Administer medications PRN for agitation or anxiety.
    - Ensure safety in the physical environment (a lowered bed, removal of scatter rugs to prevent falls).
    - Provide compensatory memory aids (clocks, calendars, photographs, memorabilia, seasonal decorations, familiar objects). Reorient as necessary.
    - Provide eyeglasses and assistive hearing devices as needed.
    - Keep a consistent daily routine.
    - Maintain consistent caregivers.
    - Ensure adequate food and fluid intake.
    - Allow for safe pacing and wandering.
    - Cover or remove mirrors to decrease fear and agitation.
  - o Communication
    - Communicate in calm, reassuring tones.
    - Do not argue or question hallucinations or delusions.
    - Reinforce reality.

- Reinforce orientation to time, place, and person.

- Introduce self to client with each new contact.

- Establish eye contact and use short, simple sentences when speaking to clients.

- Encourage reminiscence about happy times. Talk about familiar things.

- Break instructions and activities into short timeframes.

- Limit the number of choices when dressing or eating.

- Minimize the need for decision making and abstract thinking to avoid frustration.

- Avoid confrontation.

- Encourage family visitation as appropriate.

- Medications

  ○ Medications, such as donepezil (Aricept), rivastigmine (Exelon), and galantamine (Razadyne), increase acetylcholine at cholinergic synapses by inhibiting its breakdown by acetylcholinesterase, which increases the availability of acetylcholine at neurotransmitter receptor sites in the CNS.

    - Therapeutic uses of these medications include the client's improved ability to perform self-care and slow cognitive deterioration of Alzheimer's disease for clients who have mild to moderate Alzheimer's dementia.

SIDE/ADVERSE EFFECTS	NURSING INTERVENTIONS/CLIENT EDUCATION
Nausea and diarrhea, which occur in approximately 10% of clients	• Monitor for gastrointestinal side effects and for fluid volume deficits. • Promote adequate fluid intake. • The provider may titrate the dosage to reduce symptoms.
Bradycardia	• Tell families to monitor pulse rate for clients who live at home. • Clients should be screened for underlying heart disease.

- Contraindications/precautions

  □ Use cholinesterase inhibitors with caution in clients who have pre-existing asthma or other obstructive pulmonary disorders. Bronchoconstriction may be caused by an increase of acetylcholine.

MEDICATION/FOOD INTERACTIONS	NURSING INTERVENTIONS/CLIENT EDUCATION
Concurrent use of NSAIDs (aspirin) may cause gastrointestinal bleeding.	• Ask about the use of over-the-counter NSAIDs. • Monitor for clinical manifestations of gastrointestinal bleeding.
Antihistamines, tricyclic antidepressants, and conventional antipsychotics (medications that block cholinergic receptors) can reduce the therapeutic effects of donepezil.	• Use of cholinergic receptor blocking medications for clients taking any cholinesterase inhibitor is not recommended.

- Nursing Considerations
  - Start dosage low and gradually increase until side effects are no longer tolerable or medication is no longer beneficial.
  - Monitor for adverse effects and reinforce education for clients and families about these effects. Taper medication when discontinuing to prevent abrupt progression of symptoms.
  - Monitor clients for the ability to swallow tablets. Most of the medications are available in tablets and oral solutions. Donepezil is available in an orally disintegrating tablet.
  - Administer with or without food.
  - Donepezil has a long half-life and is administered once daily at bedtime. The other cholinesterase inhibitors are usually administered twice daily.
- Medications, such as memantine (Namenda), block the entry of calcium into nerve cells, thus slowing down brain-cell death.
  - Memantine is the only medication approved for moderate to severe stages of Alzheimer's disease.
  - Nursing Considerations
    - Memantine may be used concurrently with a cholinesterase inhibitor.
    - Administer the medication with or without food.
    - Monitor for common side effects, including dizziness, headache, confusion, and constipation.

- Alternative/Complementary Therapies
  - Estrogen therapy for women may prevent Alzheimer's disease, but it is not useful in decreasing the effects of pre-existing dementia.
  - Ginkgo biloba, an herbal product, is used by some clients to aid their memory. Instruct clients to inform the provider of the use of ginkgo biloba due to potential interactions, such as the risk for bleeding in clients taking antiplatelet medications, as well as the risk for seizures in clients taking medications that may lower seizure threshold.

- Care After Discharge
  - Educate family/caregivers about the client's illness, methods of care, and adaptation of the home environment.
  - Ensure a safe environment in the home. Questions to ask include:
    - Will the client wander out into the street if doors are left unlocked?
    - Is the client able to remember his address and name?
    - Does the client harm others when allowed to wander in a long-term care facility?
  - Implement home safety measures.
    - Remove scatter rugs.
    - Install door locks that cannot be easily opened.

- ■ Lock water heater thermostat and turning water temperature down to a safe level.

- ■ Provide good lighting, especially on stairs.

- ■ Install handrails on stairs and mark step edges with colored tape.

- ■ Place mattresses on the floor.

- ■ Remove clutter, keeping clear, wide pathways for walking through a room.

- ■ Secure electrical cords to baseboards.

- ■ Store cleaning supplies in locked cupboards.

- ■ Install handrails in bathrooms.

  - ○ Monitor for improvement in memory and the client's quality of life.

- • Support for Caregivers

  - ○ Determine learning needs for the client and especially the client's family members as the client's cognitive ability progressively declines.

  - ○ Review the resources available to the family as the client's health declines. Include long-term care options. A wide variety of home care and community resources may be available to the family in many areas of the country, and these resources may allow the client to remain at home, rather than in an institution.

  - ○ Provide support for caregivers. Recommend local support groups for caregivers, as well as respite care.

  - ○ Establish a routine. Make sure all caregivers know and apply the routine. Attempt to have consistency in caregivers.

- • Client Outcomes

  - ○ The client will demonstrate improvement in cognition, memory, and ability to perform self-care.

  - ○ The client will remain free from injury.

Ⓐ APPLICATION EXERCISES

Scenario: An older adult client has just been diagnosed with stage 4 Alzheimer's disease. He is experiencing short-term memory loss, and his wife has quit her job to stay home with him because he is depressed and is also distressed about being so forgetful. The client just began wearing a transdermal rivastigmine (Exelon) patch.

1. How does rivastigmine (Exelon) work, and what are the benefits of the medication for this client?

2. The client's wife asks what side effects of rivastigmine she should watch for. How should the nurse reply?

3. The client's wife asks the nurse about using gingko biloba to treat her husband's Alzheimer's disease. What information should the nurse give her?

4. A client who has moderately severe dementia is admitted to a long-term care facility. Which of the following findings should the nurse expect? (Select all that apply.)

   _____ No change in level of consciousness

   _____ Stable vital signs

   _____ Daily changes in behavior

   _____ Restlessness

   _____ Disorientation

APPLICATION EXERCISES ANSWER KEY

Scenario: An older adult client has just been diagnosed with stage 4 Alzheimer's disease. He is experiencing short-term memory loss, and his wife has quit her job to stay home with him because he is depressed and is also distressed about being so forgetful. The client just began wearing a transdermal rivastigmine (Exelon) patch.

1. How does rivastigmine (Exelon) work, and what are the benefits of the medication for this client?

   Cholinesterase inhibitors prevent the breakdown of acetylcholine in cerebral neurons, increasing its availability in the brain. Rivastigmine and the other cholinesterase inhibitors slow memory loss and improve behavior and daily function. Their use slows the progression of the disease for a few months.

 NCLEX® Connection: Pharmacological Therapies, Expected Effects/Outcomes

2. The client's wife asks what side effects of rivastigmine she should watch for. How should the nurse reply?

   The most common adverse effects of rivastigmine are nausea and vomiting. She should watch for these and also monitor the client's heart rate, as this medication can cause bradycardia.

 NCLEX® Connection: Pharmacological Therapies, Adverse Effects/Contraindications/Side Effects/Interactions

3. The client's wife asks the nurse about using gingko biloba to treat her husband's Alzheimer's disease. What information should the nurse give her?

   Some studies have shown that gingko biloba is able to stabilize or improve cognitive function briefly in clients with Alzheimer's disease (mild stage; not effective in late or severe states). Like the cholinesterase-inhibiting medications, it does not cure the disease. It may, however, slow progression for a few months. Gingko biloba has antiplatelet activity that may increase the risk of bleeding, especially if given with aspirin or anticoagulants.

 NCLEX® Connection: Pharmacological Therapies, Expected Actions/Outcomes

4. A client who has moderately severe dementia is admitted to a long-term care facility. Which of the following findings should the nurse expect? (Select all that apply.)

__X__ **No change in level of consciousness**

__X__ **Stable vital signs**

_____ Daily changes in behavior

__X__ **Restlessness**

__X__ **Disorientation**

Unless there is an underlying medical disorder, clients who have dementia will likely have no changes in level of consciousness or vital signs. Behavioral changes are gradual with dementia and are unlikely to shift on a daily basis. Clients who have dementia in moderate to advanced stages are typically restless and disoriented to time, place, and person.

Ⓝ NCLEX® Connection: Psychosocial Integrity, Physiological Adaptations, Basic Pathophysiology

| UNIT 3 | PSYCHOBIOLOGIC DISORDERS |
| Chapter 16 | Substance and Other Dependencies |

Overview

- The various substance abuse and dependence disorders recognized and defined by the DSM-IV-TR include the following:

  o Substance abuse – Involves a repeated use of chemical substances, leading to clinically significant impairment over a 12-month period, and at least one of the following problems:

    ▪ Inability to perform normal duties at home, school, or work

    ▪ Taking part in hazardous situations or risky behaviors while impaired (driving)

    ▪ Repeated legal or other personal problems caused by the substance use (losing one's job due to missed work time)

    ▪ Continued use of the substance, despite the problems it has caused

  o Substance dependence – Involves repeated use of chemical substances, leading to clinically significant impairment over a 12-month period, and three or more of the following:

    ▪ The presence of tolerance – A need for higher and higher doses of a substance to achieve the desired effect (requiring larger amounts of alcohol to feel euphoric)

    ▪ The phenomenon of withdrawal – The stopping or reduction of intake that results in specific physical and psychological clinical manifestations (tremors and headaches when the substance is not available)

    ▪ The substance taken in larger amounts or for longer periods than intended (continuing to take a prescribed opioid after surgical pain has ceased)

    ▪ A persistent (but unsuccessful) desire to control use of the substance

    ▪ Progressively more time spent in obtaining, using, and recovering from use of the substance

    ▪ Reduction in normal social or occupational activities

    ▪ Continued use in the presence of related physical or psychological problems that are acknowledged by clients

  o Non-substance related dependency (process addictions) – Dependence is on a behavior. Examples:

    ▪ Gambling

    ▪ Sexual behaviors

- Shopping or spending
- Internet use

- Addiction is characterized by:

  o Loss of control due to participation in the dependency, whether that dependency is on a substance or to a process

  o Participation in the dependency despite continuing associated problems

  o A tendency to relapse back into the dependency

- The defense mechanism of denial is commonly used by clients who have problems with drug abuse or dependency. For example, a person with long-term nicotine abuse might say, "I can quit whenever I want to, but smoking really doesn't cause me any problems." Frequently, denial prevents a client from obtaining help with substance or process abuse or dependency.

Data Collection

- Risk Factors

  o Genetics – Predisposition to developing a dependency disorder due to family history

  o Lowered self-esteem

  o Lowered tolerance for pain and frustration

  o Few meaningful personal relationships

  o Few life successes

  o Risk-taking tendencies

  o Sociocultural theories

    - Certain cultures within the United States, such as Native American groups, have a high percentage of members with alcohol dependence. Other cultures, such as Asian groups, have a low percentage of alcohol dependence.

    - Peer pressure and other sociologic factors can increase the likelihood of substance use.

  o Older adult clients may have a history of alcohol abuse or may develop a pattern of alcohol or substance abuse later in life due to life stressors (losing a spouse or a friend, retirement, social isolation).

- Subjective and Objective Data

  o The nursing history should include the following:

    - Type of substance or compulsive behavior

    - Pattern and frequency of substance use

    - Amount of substance used

    - Age at onset of substance abuse

- Changes in use patterns
- Periods of abstinence in history
- Previous withdrawal symptoms
- Date of last substance use/compulsive behavior
- Review of systems
  □ Blackout or loss of consciousness
  □ Changes in bowel movements
  □ Weight loss or weight gain
  □ Experience of stressful situation
  □ Sleep problems
  □ Chronic pain
  □ Concern over substance abuse
  □ Cutting down on consumption or behavior

- Older adult clients
  - Alcohol use can lead to falls and other injuries, memory loss, somatic reports (headaches), and changes in sleep patterns.
  - Alcohol dependence may include a decrease in ability for self-care (functional status), urinary incontinence, and signs of dementia.
  - Older adults may show clinical manifestations of alcohol abuse at lower doses than younger adults.
  - Exposure to multiple medications in addition to age-related physiological changes raises the likelihood of adverse effects, such as confusion and falls.

- Central Nervous System Depressants
  - CNS depressants can produce physiological and psychological dependence and may have cross-tolerance, cross-dependency, and an additive effect when taken concurrently.

INTENDED EFFECTS	TOXIC EFFECTS	WITHDRAWAL SIGNS/SYMPTOMS
Alcohol (ethanol)		
• Relaxation • Decreased social anxiety • Maintaining calm	• A laboratory blood alcohol concentration (BAC) of 0.08% is considered legally intoxicated for adults operating automobiles in every U.S. state. The level may be lower for different groups (adolescents younger than 18 years old). Death could occur from acute toxicity in levels greater than about 0.35%. o BAC depends on many factors, including body weight, gender, concentration of alcohol in drinks, number of drinks, gastric absorption rate, and the individual's tolerance level. • Effects of excess – Altered judgment, decreased motor skills, decreased level of consciousness (which can include stupor or coma), respiratory arrest, peripheral collapse, and death (can occur with large doses) • Chronic use – Direct cardiovascular damage, liver damage (ranging from fatty liver to cirrhosis), erosive gastritis and GI bleeding, acute pancreatitis, and sexual dysfunction	• Effects usually start within 4 to 12 hr of the last intake of alcohol, peak after 24 to 48 hr, and then subside. • Clinical findings include abdominal cramping, vomiting, tremors, restlessness and inability to sleep, increased heart rate, blood pressure, respiratory rate, temperature, and tonic-clonic seizures. • Alcohol withdrawal delirium may occur 2 to 3 days after cessation of alcohol and may last 2 to 3 days. This is considered a medical emergency. Clinical manifestations include severe disorientation, psychotic symptoms (hallucinations), severe hypertension, cardiac dysrhythmias, and delirium. Clinical findings may progress to death.

INTENDED EFFECTS	TOXIC EFFECTS	WITHDRAWAL SIGNS/SYMPTOMS
Benzodiazepines (diazepam [Valium]) can be taken orally or injected.		
• Decreased anxiety • Sedation	• Increased drowsiness and sedation, agitation, disorientation, nausea, and vomiting • Respiratory depression • An antidote, flumazenil (Romazicon), available for IV use for benzodiazepine toxicity • Rapid dependence	• Anxiety, insomnia, diaphoresis, hypertension, possible psychotic reactions, and sometimes seizure activity
Barbiturates (pentobarbital [Nembutal], secobarbital [Seconal]) can be taken orally or injected.		
• Sedation • Decreased anxiety	• Respiratory depression and decreased level of consciousness, which may be fatal • No antidote to reverse barbiturate toxicity	• Milder symptoms – The same as those seen in alcohol withdrawal • Severe symptoms – Life-threatening convulsions, delirium, and cardiovascular collapse similar to that of alcohol withdrawal
Cannabis (marijuana, hashish [more potent]) can be smoked or eaten.		
• Euphoria, sedation • Hallucinations, • Decrease of nausea and vomiting secondary to chemotherapy • Management of chronic pain • Focus only on one task	• Chronic use – Lung cancer, chronic bronchitis, and other respiratory effects • In high doses, occurrence of paranoia (delusions, hallucinations)	• Some depression

- Central Nervous System Stimulants

    ○ The CNS stimulation seen in specific CNS stimulants is dependent on the area of the brain and spinal cord affected.

INTENDED EFFECTS	TOXIC EFFECTS	WITHDRAWAL SIGNS/SYMPTOMS
Cocaine can be inhaled (snorted), smoked, or injected.		
• Rush of euphoria and pleasure • Increased energy	• Mild toxicity – Dizziness, irritability, tremor, and blurred vision • Severe effects – Hallucinations, seizures, extreme fever, tachycardia, hypertension, chest pain, possible cardiovascular collapse, and death	• Characteristic withdrawal syndrome occurs within 1 hr to several days of cessation of drug use. • Depression, fatigue, craving, excess sleeping or insomnia, dramatic unpleasant dreams, and psychomotor retardation or agitation • Not life threatening, but possible occurrence of suicidal ideation
Amphetamines can be taken orally, smoked, or injected.		
• Increased energy • Euphoria similar to cocaine	• Impaired judgment, psychomotor agitation, hypervigilance, and extreme irritability • Acute cardiovascular effects (tachycardia, elevated blood pressure), which could cause death	• Craving, depression, fatigue, and sleeping (similar to those of cocaine) • Not life threatening
Nicotine can be inhaled (cigarettes, cigars), or snuffed or chewed (smokeless tobacco).		
• Relaxation • Decreased anxiety	• Highly toxic, but acute toxicity seen only in children or when exposure is to nicotine in pesticides • Also contains other harmful chemicals that are highly toxic and have long-term effects • Long-term effects – Cardiovascular disease (hypertension, stroke) and respiratory disease (emphysema, lung cancer); with smokeless tobacco, irritation to oral mucous membranes and cancer	• Abstinence syndrome is evidenced by irritability, craving, nervousness, restlessness, anxiety, insomnia, increased appetite, and difficulty concentrating.

INTENDED EFFECTS	TOXIC EFFECTS	WITHDRAWAL SIGNS/SYMPTOMS
Opioids (heroin, morphine, hydromorphone [Dilaudid]) can be injected, inhaled, or smoked.		
• A rush of euphoria (extreme well-being) • Relief from pain	• Decreased respirations and level of consciousness, which may cause death • An antidote, naloxone (Narcan), available for IV use to relieve symptoms of overdose	• Abstinence syndrome begins with sweating and rhinorrhea progressing to piloerection (gooseflesh), tremors, and irritability followed by severe weakness, nausea and vomiting, pain in the muscles and bones, and muscle spasms. • Withdrawal is very unpleasant but not life-threatening, and it is self-limiting to 7 to 10 days.
Inhalants (amyl nitrate, nitrous oxide, solvents) are "sniffed," "huffed," or "bagged," often by young children or teenagers.		
• Euphoria	• Depends on the drug, but generally can cause CNS depression, clinical findings of psychosis (hallucinations), respiratory depression, and possible death	• None
Hallucinogens (lysergic acid diethylamide [LSD], mescaline [peyote], phencyclidine piperidine [PCP]) can be taken orally, injected, or smoked.		
• Heightened sense of self and altered perceptions (colors being more vivid while under the influence)	• Panic attacks and flashbacks (visual disturbances or hallucinations), which can occur intermittently for years	• None

- Illegal drugs continue to increase in potency, which increases the risk for onset of mental illness and major medical problems.

- Standardized Screening Tools

   o Michigan Alcohol Screening Test (MAST) or Michigan Alcohol Screening Test – Geriatric (MAST-G)

   o Addiction Severity Index

   o Recovery Attitude and Treatment Evaluator

- Brief Drug Abuse Screen Test
- CAGE-AID – This screening tool asks questions of clients to determine how clients perceive their current substance use.

Collaborative Care

- Nursing Care
    - Perform self-assessment regarding feelings related to abuses, as those feelings may be transferred to clients through body language and the terminology used in communicating with clients. An objective, nonjudgmental approach by nurses is imperative.
    - Use open-ended questions, such as "When was your last drink?"
    - Focus on safety during the acute stage of abuse.
        - Maintain a safe environment to prevent falls; implement seizure precautions as necessary.
        - Provide close observation for withdrawal symptoms, possibly one-on-one supervision. Physical restraint should be a last resort.
        - Orient clients to time, place, and person.
        - Maintain adequate nutrition and fluid balance.
        - Create a low-stimulation environment.
        - Administer withdrawal medications as prescribed.
        - Monitor for covert substance abuse during the detoxification period.
    - Provide emotional support and reassurance to clients and their families.
        - Reinforce teaching with clients and families about codependent behaviors.
    - Begin to instruct clients and families about addiction and the initial treatment goal of abstinence.
    - Tell clients and families to remove prescription medications in the home that are not being used. Encourage clients not to share medication with someone for whom that medication is not prescribed.
    - Begin to develop motivation and commitment for abstinence and recovery (abstinence plus working a program of personal growth and self-discovery).
    - Encourage self-responsibility.
    - Help clients develop an emergency plan – A list of things clients would need to do and people they would need to contact.
    - Encourage attendance at self-help groups.

- Interdisciplinary Care

  o Dual diagnosis, or comorbidity, means that an individual has both a mental illness (depression) and a problem with substance or process abuse. Treat both disorders simultaneously, using a team approach.

  o Individual psychotherapies

    ▪ Use cognitive behavioral therapies, such as relaxation techniques or cognitive reframing, to decrease anxiety and change behavior.

  o Group therapy

    ▪ Have groups of clients with similar diagnoses meet in an outpatient setting or within mental health residential facilities.

  o Family therapy

    ▪ This therapy identifies codependency, which is a common behavior demonstrated by the significant other, family, and friends of an individual with substance or process dependency, and assists the family to change that behavior. The codependent person reacts in over-responsible ways that actually allow the dependent individual to continue the substance (or process) abuse or dependency. For example, a spouse may call the client's employer with an excuse of illness when the client is actually intoxicated.

    ▪ Reinforce teaching to families about abuse of specific substances.

    ▪ Provide clients and families with information about issues such as family coping, problem solving, relapse signs, and availability of support groups.

- Pharmacological Therapy

  o Medications

    ▪ Alcohol withdrawal – Diazepam (Valium), lorazepam (Ativan), chlordiazepoxide (Librium), carbamazepine (Tegretol), and clonidine (Catapres)

    ▪ Alcohol abstinence – Disulfiram (Antabuse), naltrexone (ReVia), and acamprosate (Campral)

    ▪ Opioid withdrawal – Methadone (Dolophine) substitution, clonidine (Catapres), buprenorphine (Subutex), and buprenorphine combined with naloxone (Suboxone)

    ▪ Nicotine withdrawal – Bupropion (Wellbutrin) and nicotine replacement therapy (nicotine gum [Nicorette], nicotine patch [Nicotrol])

    ▪ Nursing Considerations

      □ Monitor the client's vital signs and neurological status.

      □ Provide for client safety by implementing seizure precautions.

- Client Education

  □ Encourage clients to adhere to the treatment plan by participating in the plan of care.

  □ Advise clients taking disulfiram (Antabuse) to avoid all alcohol, as drinking while taking disulfiram can lead to neurological and gastrointestinal complications.

- Care After Discharge

  o Client Education

    - Reinforce teaching with clients about how to recognize signs and symptoms of relapse and factors that contribute to relapse.

    - Reinforce teaching about cognitive-behavioral techniques to help maintain sobriety and to create feelings of pleasure from activities other than using substances or from process addictions.

    - Assist clients to develop communication skills to communicate with coworkers and family members while sober.

    - Encourage clients and their families to attend a 12-step program, such as Alcoholics Anonymous (AA), Narcotics Anonymous, Gamblers Anonymous, and family groups like Al-Anon or Alateen.

      □ These programs will teach clients the following:

        ▸ Abstinence is necessary for recovery.

        ▸ A higher power is needed to assist in recovery.

        ▸ They are not responsible for their disease but are responsible for their recovery.

        ▸ Others cannot be blamed for their addictions, and they must acknowledge their feelings and problems.

- Client Outcomes

  o The client will verbalize coping strategies to use in times of stress.

  o The client will remain substance free.

  o The client will remain free from injury.

  o The client will attend a 12-step program regularly.

Ⓐ APPLICATION EXERCISES

Scenario: A 45-year-old client was admitted to an acute-care facility for medically supervised detoxification 8 hr ago. The client was admitted because he was involved in a motor-vehicle crash while driving under the influence of alcohol. Data collection indicates no physical injury, a blood alcohol concentration (BAC) of 200 g/dL (0.20%), and a 30-year history of alcohol abuse. He has been in rehabilitation facilities several times but has always relapsed. He lives alone after a separation from his wife and three teenage children, whom the client has not seen in a year. The client has not been able to keep a job due to poor attendance, and he has been out of work for the past 6 months. The client also has additional driving under the influence (DUI) citations.

1. According to the DSM-IV-TR, which signs of substance dependence does this client have?

2. When collecting data from a client who has alcohol withdrawal, which of the following observations should the nurse expect to make? (Select all that apply.)

   _____ Bradycardia

   _____ Respiratory depression

   _____ Hypotension

   _____ Abdominal cramping

   _____ Restlessness

3. Which of the following interventions is the highest priority for the client at this time?

   A. Create a low-stimulation environment.

   B. Monitor for covert substance abuse.

   C. Implement seizure precautions.

   D. Encourage participation in group therapy sessions.

4. Which of the following medications should the nurse anticipate administering to help clients maintain their abstinence from alcohol?

   A. Lorazepam (Ativan)

   B. Bupropion (Wellbutrin)

   C. Disulfiram (Antabuse)

   D. Clonidine (Catapres)

5. Which of the following is an adverse effect of hallucinogens, such as lysergic acid diethylamide (LSD) and phencyclidine piperidine (PCP)?

   A. Panic attacks

   B. Hypothermia

   C. Constricted pupils

   D. Muscle flaccidity

(A) **APPLICATION EXERCISES ANSWER KEY**

Scenario: A 45-year-old client was admitted to an acute-care facility for medically supervised detoxification 8 hr ago. The client was admitted because he was involved in a motor-vehicle crash while driving under the influence of alcohol. Data collection indicates no physical injury, a blood alcohol concentration (BAC) of 200 g/dL (0.20%), and a 30-year history of alcohol abuse. He has been in rehabilitation facilities several times but has always relapsed. He lives alone after a separation from his wife and three teenage children, whom the client has not seen in a year. The client has not been able to keep a job due to poor attendance, and he has been out of work for the past 6 months. The client also has additional driving under the influence (DUI) citations.

1. According to the DSM-IV-TR, which signs of substance dependence does this client have?

   Beginning to experience withdrawal symptoms

   Several attempts to stop drinking with subsequent relapses

   Reduction in usual social or occupational activities – has lost his family and his job

   Continued use of the substance despite the problems it has caused

(N) NCLEX® Connection: Psychosocial Integrity, Chemical and Other Dependencies

2. When collecting data from a client who has alcohol withdrawal, which of the following observations should the nurse expect to make? (Select all that apply.)

_____	Bradycardia
_____	Respiratory depression
_____	Hypotension
__X__	**Abdominal cramping**
__X__	**Restlessness**

   Abdominal cramping, restlessness, an increased respiratory rate, inability to sleep, depressed mood, and irritability are all expected findings for a client who is withdrawing from alcohol. Tachycardia and hypertension are common, not bradycardia and hypotension.

(N) NCLEX® Connection: Psychosocial Integrity, Chemical and Other Dependencies

3. Which of the following interventions is the highest priority for the client at this time?

    A. Create a low-stimulation environment.

    B. Monitor for covert substance abuse.

    C. Implement seizure precautions.

    D. Encourage participation in group therapy sessions.

    The greatest risk to the client at this time is injury from seizures and falls. Therefore, implementing seizure precautions is the highest priority to prevent injury in the event of a seizure. Reducing environmental stimulation, monitoring for any substance abuse, and encouraging participation in group therapy sessions are all important but are not the highest priority at this time.

 NCLEX® Connection: Safety and Infection Control, Accident/Error/Injury Prevention

4. Which of the following medications should the nurse anticipate administering to help clients maintain their abstinence from alcohol?

    A. Lorazepam (Ativan)

    B. Bupropion (Wellbutrin)

    C. Disulfiram (Antabuse)

    D. Clonidine (Catapres)

    Disulfiram helps clients maintain abstinence from alcohol. Clients who drink alcohol while taking disulfiram might have a mild reaction, such as nausea and vomiting, or a more severe reaction that can lead to respiratory depression and death. Lorazepam is administered for acute alcohol withdrawal. Bupropion is administered for nicotine withdrawal. Clonidine is administered for opioid withdrawal.

 NCLEX® Connection: Pharmacological Therapies, Expected Effects/Outcomes

5. Which of the following is an adverse effect of hallucinogens, such as lysergic acid diethylamide (LSD) and phencyclidine piperidine (PCP)?

    A. Panic attacks

    B. Hypothermia

    C. Constricted pupils

    D. Muscle flaccidity

    After ingestion of hallucinogens, panic attacks and flashbacks (visual disturbances or hallucinations) can recur for years. Increases in temperature, heart rate, and respiratory rate are common with hallucinogen use. Dilated pupils and muscle rigidity are also common with hallucinogen use.

 NCLEX® Connection: Psychosocial Integrity, Chemical and Other Dependencies

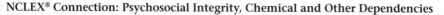

UNIT 3	PSYCHOBIOLOGIC DISORDERS
Chapter 17	Eating Disorders

Overview

- The various eating disorders recognized and defined by the DSM-IV-TR include the following:

  o Anorexia nervosa

    ▪ Clients are preoccupied with food and the rituals of eating, along with a voluntary refusal to eat.

    ▪ Clients exhibit a morbid fear of obesity and a refusal to maintain a minimally normal body weight (less than 85% of expected normal weight for the individual) in the absence of a physical cause.

    ▪ Clients have a body image disturbance.

    ▪ This disorder occurs most often in females from adolescence to young adulthood. Only 5% to 10% of clients who have anorexia nervosa are male.

    ▪ Two types:

      □ Restricting type – The individual drastically restricts food intake and does not binge or purge.

      □ Binge-eating/purging type – The individual engages in binge eating or purging behaviors.

  o Bulimia nervosa

    ▪ Clients recurrently eat large quantities of food over a short period of time (bingeing), which may be followed by inappropriate compensatory behaviors, such as self-induced vomiting (purging), to rid the body of the excess calories.

    ▪ Most clients who have bulimia maintain a weight within a normal range or slightly higher.

    ▪ The average age of onset in females is 15 to 18 years of age.

    ▪ About 10% to 15% of clients who have bulimia are males. For males, onset generally occurs between 18 and 26 years of age, and bingeing with the use of excessive exercise (nonpurging type) is most common.

    ▪ Two types:

      □ Purging type – Clients use self-induced vomiting, laxatives, diuretics, and/or enemas to lose or maintain weight.

      □ Nonpurging type – Clients may also compensate for bingeing through other means, such as excessive exercise and misuse of laxatives, diuretics, and/or enemas.

- Mortality rate for eating disorders is high, and suicide is also a risk.

- Treatment modalities focus on normalizing eating patterns and beginning to address the issues raised by the illness.

- Comorbidities include major depressive disorder and dysthymia (50% - 75%), obsessive compulsive disorder, substance abuse, and anxiety disorders.

Data Collection

- Risk Factors

  ○ Females

    ▪ Family genetics – More commonly seen in families with sisters and mothers with eating disorders

    ▪ Biological – Hypothalamic, neurotransmitter, hormonal, or biochemical imbalance, with disturbances of the serotonin neurotransmitter pathways seeming to be implicated

    ▪ Interpersonal relationships – Influenced by parental pressure and the need to succeed

    ▪ Psychological influences – Rigidity and ritualism; separation and individuation conflicts; feelings of ineffectiveness, helplessness, and depression; and distorted body image

    ▪ Environmental factors – Pressure from society to have the "perfect body," culture of abundance

    ▪ Individual history of being a "picky" eater in childhood

    ▪ Participation in athletics, especially at an elite level of competition

  ○ Males

    ▪ Participation in a sport where lean body build is prized (bicycling) or where a specific weight is necessary (wrestling)

    ▪ A history of obesity

- Subjective and Objective Data

  ○ Nursing history should include the following:

    ▪ The client's perception of the issue

    ▪ Eating habits

    ▪ History of dieting

    ▪ Methods of weight control (restricting, purging, exercising)

    ▪ Value attached to a specific shape and weight

    ▪ Interpersonal and social functioning

    ▪ Difficulty with impulsivity, as well as compulsivity

    ▪ Family and interpersonal relationships (frequently troublesome and chaotic, reflecting a lack of nurturing)

OBJECTIVE DATA	FINDINGS
Mental status	<ul><li>Cognitive distortions include:<ul><li>Overgeneralizations – "Other girls don't like me because I'm fat."</li><li>All-or-nothing thinking – "If I eat any dessert, I'll gain 50 pounds."</li><li>Catastrophizing – "My life is over if I gain weight."</li><li>Personalization – "When I walk through the hospital hallway, I know everyone is looking at me."</li><li>Emotional reasoning – "I know I look bad because I feel bloated."</li></ul></li><li>Clients demonstrate high interest in preparing food, but not eating.</li><li>Clients are terrified of gaining weight.</li><li>The client's perception is that she is severely overweight and sees this image reflected in the mirror.</li><li>Clients may exhibit low self-esteem, impulsivity, and difficulty with interpersonal relationships.</li><li>Clients may participate in an intense physical regimen.</li></ul>
Vital signs	<ul><li>Low blood pressure with possible orthostatic hypotension</li><li>Decreased pulse and body temperature</li></ul>
Weight	<ul><li>Clients who have anorexia have a body weight that is less than 85% of expected normal weight.</li><li>Most clients who have bulimia maintain a weight within the normal range or slightly higher.</li></ul>
Skin, hair, and nails	<ul><li>Clients who have anorexia may have fine, downy hair (lanugo) on the face and back; yellowed skin; mottled, cool extremities; and poor skin turgor.</li></ul>
Head, neck, mouth, and throat	<ul><li>Clients who have bulimia may have enlargement of the parotid glands; dental erosion, and caries (if the client is purging).</li></ul>
Cardiovascular system	<ul><li>Clients who have bulimia may have irregular heart rates (dysrhythmias noted on cardiac monitor), heart failure, and cardiomyopathy.</li><li>Peripheral edema may also be present in clients who have bulimia.</li></ul>
Musculoskeletal system	<ul><li>Muscle weakness</li></ul>
Gastrointestinal system	<ul><li>Constipation</li><li>Self-induced vomiting</li><li>Excessive use of diuretics or laxatives</li></ul>
Reproductive status	<ul><li>Anorexia is accompanied by amenorrhea for at least three consecutive cycles.</li></ul>
Nutritional status	<ul><li>Electrolyte imbalances and severe dehydration</li></ul>

- ○ Criteria for inpatient treatment includes:
  - Rapid weight loss or weight loss of greater than 30% of body weight over 6 months
  - Unsuccessful weight gain in outpatient treatment or failure to adhere to treatment contract
  - Vital signs demonstrating heart rate less than 40 bpm, systolic blood pressure less than 70 mm Hg, body temperature less than 36° C (96.8° F)
  - ECG changes
  - Electrolyte disturbances
  - Severe depression
  - Suicidal behavior
  - Family crisis
- ○ Laboratory and Diagnostic Tests
  - Common laboratory abnormalities associated with anorexia include:
    - □ Hypokalemia, especially for those who are also bulimic
      - ‣ There is a direct loss of potassium due to purging (vomiting).
      - ‣ Dehydration stimulates increased aldosterone production, which leads to sodium and water retention and potassium excretion.
    - □ Anemia and leukopenia with lymphocytosis
    - □ Possible impaired liver function, shown by increased enzyme levels
    - □ Possible elevated cholesterol
    - □ Abnormal thyroid function tests
    - □ Elevated carotene levels, which cause skin to appear yellow
    - □ Decreased bone density (possible osteoporosis)
    - □ Abnormal blood glucose level
    - □ ECG changes
  - Electrolyte imbalances associated with bulimia are common and may depend on the client's method of purging (laxatives, diuretics, vomiting). Laboratory abnormalities include:
    - □ Hypokalemia
    - □ Hyponatremia
    - □ Hypochloremia
- ○ Standardized screening tools
  - Eating Disorders Inventory
  - Body Attitude Test
  - Diagnostic Survey for Eating Disorders

Collaborative Care

- Nursing Care

    o Provide a highly structured milieu in an inpatient eating disorder unit for clients requiring intensive therapy.

    o Develop and maintain a trusting nurse-client relationship through consistency and therapeutic communication.

    o Use a positive approach and support to promote clients' self-esteem and positive self-image.

    o Encourage clients to make decisions and participate in the plan of care to allow for a sense of control.

    o Establish realistic goals for weight gain.

    o Promote cognitive-behavioral therapies.

        ▪ Cognitive reframing

        ▪ Relaxation techniques

        ▪ Journal writing

        ▪ Desensitization exercises

    o Monitor the client's vital signs, I&O, and weight.

    o Use behavioral contracts to modify the client's behaviors.

    o Reward clients for positive behaviors (completing meals, consuming a set number of calories).

    o Closely monitor clients during and after meals to prevent purging, which may necessitate accompanying the client to the bathroom.

    o Monitor clients for maintenance of appropriate exercise.

    o Reinforce teaching about self-care activities.

    o Provide nutrition education to include correcting misinformation regarding food, meal planning, and food selection.

        ▪ Consider the client's preferences and ability to consume food when developing the initial eating plan.

        ▪ Establish a structured and inflexible eating schedule at the start of therapy, only permitting food during scheduled times.

        ▪ Provide small, frequent meals, which are better tolerated and will help prevent the client from feeling overwhelmed.

        ▪ Provide a diet high in fiber to control constipation.

        ▪ Provide a diet low in sodium to control fluid retention.

        ▪ Limit high-fat and gassy foods during the start of treatment.

        ▪ Administer a multivitamin and mineral supplement.

        ▪ Instruct clients to avoid caffeine.

- ○ Make arrangements for clients to attend individual, group, and family therapy to assist in resolving personal issues contributing to the eating disorder.

- Medications

  - ○ Selective serotonin reuptake inhibitors (SSRIs), such as fluoxetine (Prozac)

    - ■ Client Education

      - □ Instruct clients that medication may take 1 to 3 weeks for initial response, with up to 2 months for maximal response.

      - □ Instruct clients to avoid hazardous activities (driving, operating heavy equipment/machinery) until individual side effects are known.

      - □ Instruct clients to notify the provider if sexual dysfunction occurs and is intolerable.

- Interdisciplinary Care

  - ○ A registered dietitian should be involved to provide clients with nutritional and dietary guidance.

- Care After Discharge

  - ○ Assist clients to develop and implement a maintenance plan.

  - ○ Encourage follow-up treatment in an outpatient setting.

  - ○ Encourage client participation in a support group.

  - ○ Continue individual and family therapy as indicated.

- Client Outcomes

  - ○ The client will maintain agreed-upon weight goals.

  - ○ The client will establish normal eating habits.

  - ○ The client will verbalize a positive body image.

- Complications

  - ○ Refeeding syndrome

    - ■ Refeeding syndrome is the circulatory collapse that occurs when a client's completely compromised cardiac system is overwhelmed by a replenished vascular system after normal fluid intake resumes.

    - ■ Nursing Actions

      - □ Care for clients in a hospital setting.

      - □ Implement refeeding for at least 7 days.

      - □ Monitor serum electrolytes, and administer fluid replacement as prescribed.

  - ○ Cardiac dysrhythmias, severe bradycardia, and hypotension

    - ■ Client may be admitted to the intensive care unit until stabilized.

Ⓐ APPLICATION EXERCISES

Scenario: A nurse is working with a 16-year-old client in a community mental health facility. The client and her mother have begun exploring colleges extensively. After school, the client spends her time preparing gourmet meals for her family while her mother is working. Lately, her mother has noticed that the client is not eating the food she prepares, especially carbohydrates, and only eats small amounts of lean protein foods. Instead, she busies herself serving the rest of the family and says she is dieting in order to "have friends at college." During a recent physical examination, it was discovered that the client's weight dropped from an ideal weight for her height, 52.2 kg (115 lb), to 43.1 kg (95 lb) in the past 3 months. She has also stopped menstruating. Her provider has referred her to the mental health center for counseling.

1. List the data collection parameters that are especially important for this client.

2. Describe the types of cognitive distortions this client is demonstrating.

3. A client is hospitalized on an eating disorders unit. The client has a history of and current diagnosis of bulimia nervosa. Which of the following should the nurse expect to find? (Select all that apply.)

    _____ Hyperkalemia

    _____ Amenorrhea

    _____ ECG changes

    _____ Cool extremities

    _____ Peripheral edema

    _____ Yellowed skin

    _____ Body weight below the expected range

    _____ Tooth decay

4. A client who has bulimia has stopped vomiting on the unit and describes to the nurse feelings of being afraid of gaining weight. Which of the following is an appropriate response by the nurse?

    A. "As long as you stick to the diet you have here, you are not going to gain enough weight to worry about."

    B. "Forget about your weight for now. We are going to work on other problems while you are in the hospital."

    C. "I understand you have concerns about your weight, but tell me about your National Honor Society invitation. That's quite an accomplishment."

    D. "You are not overweight, and we'll make sure you do not become overweight. We know that is important to you."

(A) **APPLICATION EXERCISES ANSWER KEY**

Scenario: A nurse is working with a 16-year-old client in a community mental health facility. The client and her mother have begun exploring colleges extensively. After school, the client spends her time preparing gourmet meals for her family while her mother is working. Lately, her mother has noticed that the client is not eating the food she prepares, especially carbohydrates, and only eats small amounts of lean protein foods. Instead, she busies herself serving the rest of the family and says she is dieting in order to "have friends at college." During a recent physical examination, it was discovered that the client's weight dropped from an ideal weight for her height, 52.2 kg (115 lb), to 43.1 kg (95 lb) in the past 3 months. She has also stopped menstruating. Her provider has referred her to the mental health center for counseling.

1. List the data collection parameters that are especially important for this client.

    Dietary habits and history, height, weight, skin condition, vital signs, feelings about body image, and family dynamics

(N) **NCLEX® Connection: Psychosocial Integrity, Mental Health Concepts**

2. Describe the types of cognitive distortions this client is demonstrating.

    Overgeneralization (She can't make friends because others won't like her if she is fat.)

    All-or-nothing thinking (She believes that eating any carbohydrates or fats will result in unbearable weight gain.)

(N) **NCLEX® Connection: Psychosocial Integrity, Mental Health Concepts**

3. A client is hospitalized on an eating disorders unit. The client has a history of and current diagnosis of bulimia nervosa. Which of the following should the nurse expect to find? (Select all that apply.)

    _____   Hyperkalemia

    _____   Amenorrhea

    X   **ECG changes**

    _____   Cool extremities

    X   **Peripheral edema**

    _____   Yellowed skin

    _____   Body weight below the expected range

    X   **Tooth decay**

ECG changes, peripheral edema, and tooth decay are all common with bulimia nervosa. Clients who have bulimia are more likely to have weight within the expected range or slightly higher and hypokalemia. Amenorrhea, cool extremities, and yellowed skin are common with anorexia nervosa.

Ⓝ NCLEX® Connection: Psychosocial Integrity, Physiological Adaptations, Basic Pathophysiology

4. A client who has bulimia has stopped vomiting on the unit and describes to the nurse feelings of being afraid of gaining weight. Which of the following is an appropriate response by the nurse?

A. "As long as you stick to the diet you have here, you are not going to gain enough weight to worry about."

B. "Forget about your weight for now. We are going to work on other problems while you are in the hospital."

C. **"I understand you have concerns about your weight, but tell me about your National Honor Society invitation. That's quite an accomplishment."**

D. "You are not overweight, and we'll make sure you do not become overweight. We know that is important to you."

With the correct option, the nurse acknowledges the client's concerns and then focuses the conversation on the client's accomplishment. The other options minimize the client's concerns about being overweight and/or gaining weight.

Ⓝ NCLEX® Connection: Psychosocial Integrity, Psychosocial Integrity, Therapeutic Communication

UNIT 4: PSYCHOPHARMACOLOGIC THERAPIES

- Medications for Anxiety Disorders

- Medications for Depression

- Medications for Bipolar Disorders

- Medications for Psychoses

- Medications for Children and Adolescents With Mental Health Issues

- Medications for Substance Abuse

NCLEX® CONNECTIONS

When reviewing the chapters in this section, keep in mind the relevant sections of the NCLEX® outline, in particular:

CLIENT NEEDS: PHARMACOLOGICAL THERAPIES

Relevant topics/tasks include:
- Adverse Effects/Contraindications/Side Effects/Interactions
  - Reinforce client teaching on possible effects of medications .
- Expected Actions/Outcomes
  - Monitor client use of medications over time.
- Medication Administration
  - Review pertinent data prior to medication administration.

UNIT 4   PSYCHOPHARMACOLOGIC THERAPIES

Chapter 18   Medications for Anxiety Disorders

Overview

- The major medications used to treat anxiety disorders include:

  o   Benzodiazepine sedative hypnotic anxiolytics (diazepam [Valium])

  o   Atypical anxiolytic/nonbarbiturate anxiolytics (buspirone [BuSpar])

  o   Selective serotonin reuptake inhibitors (SSRIs) (paroxetine [Paxil])

- Other classifications include:

  o   Antidepressants

    ▪   Amitriptyline (Elavil), a tricyclic antidepressant (TCA)

    ▪   Phenelzine (Nardil), a monoamine oxidase inhibitor (MAOI)

    ▪   Venlafaxine (Effexor) or duloxetine (Cymbalta), both serotonin-norepinephrine reuptake inhibitors

  o   CNS stimulants (methylphenidate [Ritalin, Concerta])

  o   Sertraline (Zoloft), an SSRI

  o   Antihistamines (hydroxyzine pamoate [Vistaril])

  o   Beta blockers (propranolol [Inderal])

  o   Anticonvulsants (gabapentin [Neurontin])

MEDICATION CLASSIFICATION: BENZODIAZEPINE SEDATIVE HYPNOTIC ANXIOLYTICS

- Select Prototype Medication: diazepam (Valium)

- Other Medications:

  o   Alprazolam (Xanax)

  o   Lorazepam (Ativan)

  o   Chlordiazepoxide (Librium)

  o   Clorazepate (Tranxene)

  o   Oxazepam (Serax)

  o   Clonazepam (Klonopin)

Purpose

- Expected Pharmacological Action

    o Diazepam enhances the inhibitory effects of gamma-aminobutyric acid (GABA) in the central nervous system. Relief from anxiety occurs rapidly following administration.

- Therapeutic Uses

    o Generalized anxiety disorder (GAD) and panic disorder

    o Other uses for benzodiazepines include:

        ■ Seizure disorders

        ■ Insomnia

        ■ Muscle spasm

        ■ Alcohol withdrawal (for prevention and treatment of acute symptoms)

        ■ Induction of anesthesia

Complications

SIDE/ADVERSE EFFECTS	NURSING INTERVENTIONS/CLIENT EDUCATION
CNS depression (sedation, light-headedness, ataxia, decreased cognitive function)	• Advise clients to observe for symptoms and to notify the provider if symptoms occur. • Advise clients to avoid hazardous activities (driving, operating heavy equipment/machinery).
Anterograde amnesia – Difficulty recalling events that occur after dosing	• Advise clients to observe for symptoms and to notify the provider. Advise clients to stop the medication if symptoms occur.
Acute oral toxicity – Drowsiness, lethargy, and confusion	• Advise clients to watch for manifestations of overdose and to notify the provider if these occur. • Use gastric lavage followed by the administration of activated charcoal or saline cathartics for oral toxicity. • Monitor clients receiving flumazenil (Romazicon) by IV bolus to counteract sedation and reverse the side effects. • Assist with emergency care as necessary.
Paradoxical response (insomnia, excitation, euphoria, anxiety, rage)	• Advise clients to observe for symptoms and to notify the provider if symptoms occur.
Withdrawal symptoms (anxiety, insomnia, diaphoresis, tremors, light-headedness), which occur infrequently with short-term use	• Advise clients how to slowly taper the medication dosage after a long period of use to avoid withdrawal symptoms.

Ⓢ Contraindications/Precautions

- Diazepam is a Pregnancy Risk Category D medication.

- Benzodiazepines are classified under Schedule IV of the Controlled Substances Act.

- Diazepam is contraindicated in clients with sleep apnea and/or respiratory depression.

- Use diazepam cautiously in clients who have liver disease and/or a history of substance abuse.

Interactions

MEDICATION/FOOD INTERACTIONS	NURSING INTERVENTIONS/CLIENT EDUCATION
CNS depressants (alcohol, barbiturates, opioids) may cause respiratory depression.	• Advise clients to observe for symptoms and to notify the provider if symptoms occur. • Advise clients to avoid hazardous activities (driving, operating heavy equipment/machinery).

Nursing Administration

- Advise clients to take the medication as prescribed and to avoid abrupt discontinuation of long-term treatment to prevent withdrawal symptoms.

- Instruct clients to taper the dose over several weeks when the medication is discontinued.

- Advise clients to administer the medication with meals or snacks if GI upset occurs.

- Advise clients to swallow sustained-release tablets and to avoid chewing or crushing the tablets.

- Instruct clients about the potential for dependency during and after treatment and to notify the provider if symptoms occur.

- Medication can relieve symptoms but does not take away the stressor. Psychotherapy is important in combination with the medication.

MEDICATION CLASSIFICATION: ATYPICAL ANXIOLYTIC/ NONBARBITURATE ANXIOLYTICS

- Select Prototype Medication: buspirone (BuSpar)

Purpose

- Expected Pharmacological Action

  ○ The exact antianxiety mechanism of this medication is unknown. This medication does bind to serotonin and dopamine receptors. There is less potential for abuse than with other anxiolytics, and use of buspirone does not result in sedation or potentiate the effects of other CNS depressants.

- Therapeutic Uses

    o Panic disorder

    o Obsessive compulsive disorder (OCD)

    o Social anxiety disorder

    o Posttraumatic stress disorder (PTSD)

Complications

SIDE/ADVERSE EFFECTS	NURSING INTERVENTIONS/CLIENT EDUCATION
CNS effects include dizziness, nausea, headache, light-headedness, and agitation.	• Advise clients to take with food to decrease nausea. • Instruct clients that most side effects are self-limiting.

 Contraindications/Precautions

- Buspirone is a Pregnancy Risk Category B medication.

- Buspirone is not recommended for use by nursing mothers.

- Use buspirone cautiously in older adult clients, as well as clients with liver and/or renal dysfunction.

- Buspirone is contraindicated for concurrent use with MAOI antidepressants or for 14 days after MAOIs are discontinued. Hypertensive crisis may result.

Interactions

MEDICATION/FOOD INTERACTIONS	NURSING INTERVENTIONS/CLIENT EDUCATION
Erythromycin, ketoconazole, and grapefruit juice may increase the effects of buspirone.	• Avoid concurrent use. • Advise clients to avoid drinking grapefruit juice.

Nursing Administration

- Advise clients to take the medication with meals to prevent gastric irritation.

- Advise clients that effects do not occur immediately. It may take a week to notice first therapeutic effects, and several more weeks to reach full therapeutic benefit. Tell clients to take medication on a regular basis and not PRN.

- Instruct clients that tolerance, dependence, or withdrawal symptoms should not occur with this medication.

MEDICATION CLASSIFICATION: SELECTIVE SEROTONIN REUPTAKE INHIBITORS (SSRIS)

- Select Prototype Medication: paroxetine (Paxil)

- Other Medications:

  o Sertraline (Zoloft)

  o Escitalopram (Lexapro)

  o Fluoxetine (Prozac)

  o Fluvoxamine (Luvox)

Purpose

- Expected Pharmacological Action

  o Paroxetine selectively inhibits serotonin reuptake, allowing more serotonin to stay at the junction of the neurons.

  o It does not block uptake of dopamine or norepinephrine.

  o Paroxetine causes CNS stimulation, which can cause insomnia.

  o The medication has a long effective half-life; about 4 weeks are necessary to produce therapeutic medication levels.

- Therapeutic Uses

  o Paroxetine

    ■ Generalized anxiety disorder (GAD)

    ■ Panic disorder – Decreases both the frequency and intensity of panic attacks, and also prevents anticipatory anxiety about attacks

    ■ OCD – Reduces symptoms by increasing serotonin

    ■ Social anxiety disorder

    ■ PTSD

    ■ Depressive disorders

MEDICATION	INDICATION
Sertraline	Panic disorder, OCD, social anxiety disorder, and PTSD
Escitalopram	GAD and OCD
Fluoxetine	Panic disorder and OCD.
Fluvoxamine	OCD and social anxiety disorder

Complications

SIDE/ADVERSE EFFECTS	NURSING INTERVENTIONS/CLIENT EDUCATION
Early adverse effects (first few days/weeks) – Nausea, diaphoresis, tremor, fatigue, and drowsiness	• Advise clients that these effects should soon subside. • Instruct clients to take the medication as prescribed.
Later adverse effects (after 5 to 6 weeks of therapy) – Sexual dysfunction (impotence, delayed or absent orgasm, delayed or absent ejaculation, decreased sexual interest), weight gain, and headache	• Instruct clients to report problems with sexual function. This may be managed with dose reduction, medication holiday, and/or changing medications.
Weight gain	• Advise clients to follow a well-balanced diet and exercise regularly.
Gastrointestinal bleeding	• Advise clients to report signs of bleeding (dark stools, emesis that has the appearance of coffee grounds).
Hyponatremia – More likely in older adult clients taking diuretics	• Obtain baseline serum sodium, and monitor level periodically throughout treatment.
Serotonin syndrome • Agitation, confusion, disorientation, difficulty concentrating, anxiety, hallucinations, hyperreflexia, fever, diaphoresis, lack of coordination, and tremors • Usually begins 2 to 72 hr after initiation of treatment • Resolves when the medication is discontinued	• Watch for and advise clients to report any of these symptoms, which could indicate a lethal problem.

Bruxism – Grinding and clenching of teeth, usually during sleep	• Instruct clients to report to the provider, who may:
	  ○ Switch clients to another class of medication.
	  ○ Treat bruxism with low-dose buspirone.
	  ○ Advise clients to use a mouth guard during sleep.

Withdrawal syndrome • Nausea, sensory disturbances, anxiety, tremor, malaise, and unease • Minimized by tapering the medication slowly	• Advise clients how to slowly taper the medication dosage after a long period of use to avoid withdrawal symptoms.

Ⓢ Contraindications/Precautions

- Paroxetine is a Pregnancy Risk Category D medication. Other SSRIs pose less risk during pregnancy.

- Paroxetine is contraindicated in clients taking MAOIs.

- Clients taking paroxetine should avoid alcohol.

- Use paroxetine cautiously in clients with liver and renal dysfunction, seizure disorders, a history of gastrointestinal bleeding, or those taking NSAIDs or anticoagulants.

Interactions

MEDICATION/FOOD INTERACTIONS	NURSING INTERVENTIONS/CLIENT EDUCATION
Concurrent use of MAOIs or tricyclic antidepressants with paroxetine can cause serotonin syndrome.	• Educate clients about this combination. • Avoid concurrent use.

Nursing Administration

- Advise clients that paroxetine may be taken with food. Sleep disturbances may be minimized by taking the medication in the morning.

- Instruct clients to take the medication on a daily basis to establish therapeutic plasma levels.

- Assist clients with medication regimen adherence by informing clients that therapeutic effects may not be experienced for 1 to 3 weeks.

Nursing Evaluation of Medication Effectiveness

- Depending on therapeutic intent, effectiveness may be evidenced by:

  o Maintenance of a normal sleep pattern

  o Verbalization of feeling less anxious and more relaxed

  o Greater ability to participate in social and occupational interactions

(A) APPLICATION EXERCISES

1. A client has been prescribed diazepam (Valium) for generalized anxiety disorder. The client had originally told her provider that she took no other medications. However, before leaving the clinic, she says to the nurse, "Oh, I forgot that I do take a sleeping pill at night for insomnia, and I also drink a glass of wine before bedtime to make sure I sleep." What should be the nurse's concerns about this information, and which interventions are necessary?

2. Which of the following is an antidote for benzodiazepine overdose or toxicity?

   A. Buspirone (BuSpar)

   B. Amitriptyline (Elavil)

   C. Flumazenil (Romazicon)

   D. Naloxone (Narcan)

3. A nurse knows that a client who has just been prescribed buspirone (BuSpar) for long-term treatment of anxiety understands the instructions when she says,

   A. "I will not take the medicine with meals."

   B. "I will be able to keep taking this drug if I become pregnant."

   C. "I will not take the medicine with grapefruit juice."

   D. "I will take the medicine when I feel an anxiety attack coming on."

4. A client has been taking sertraline (Zoloft) for 3 days to treat an anxiety disorder. He calls the community mental health facility and tells the nurse that the medication has not helped him as he is still feeling anxious. How should the nurse reply?

APPLICATION EXERCISES ANSWER KEY

1. A client has been prescribed diazepam (Valium) for generalized anxiety disorder. The client had originally told her provider that she took no other medications. However, before leaving the clinic, she says to the nurse, "Oh, I forgot that I do take a sleeping pill at night for insomnia, and I also drink a glass of wine before bedtime to make sure I sleep." What should be the nurse's concerns about this information, and which interventions are necessary?

   Taking a benzodiazepine concurrently with other CNS agonists, including alcohol, can cause an overdose marked by increased sedation, lack of coordination, and confusion. The nurse should report this information to the provider before the client leaves the clinic.

   NCLEX® Connection: Pharmacological Therapies, Adverse Effects/ Contraindications/Side Effects/Interactions

2. Which of the following is an antidote for benzodiazepine overdose or toxicity?

   A. Buspirone (BuSpar)

   B. Amitriptyline (Elavil)

   C. Flumazenil (Romazicon)

   D. Naloxone (Narcan)

   Flumazenil is a benzodiazepine receptor antagonist, which specifically reverses an overdose of benzodiazepines. Buspirone is a nonbarbiturate anxiolytic, and amitriptyline is a tricyclic antidepressant. Naloxone is an opioid antagonist used to reverse an overdose of opioids, such as morphine sulfate.

   NCLEX® Connection: Pharmacological Therapies, Expected Actions/Outcomes

3. A nurse knows that a client who has just been prescribed buspirone (BuSpar) for long-term treatment of anxiety understands the instructions when she says,

   A. "I will not take the medicine with meals."

   B. "I will be able to keep taking this drug if I become pregnant."

   C. "I will not take the medicine with grapefruit juice."

   D. "I will take the medicine when I feel an anxiety attack coming on."

   Instruct clients to avoid grapefruit juice, as it can increase the effects of buspirone. Instruct clients to take with food to decrease nausea, to avoid during pregnancy, and to take on a regular basis and not PRN.

   NCLEX® Connection: Pharmacological Therapies, Medication Administration

4. A client has been taking sertraline (Zoloft) for 3 days to treat an anxiety disorder. He calls the community mental health facility and tells the nurse that the medication has not helped him as he is still feeling anxious. How should the nurse reply?

    Sertraline is a selective serotonin reuptake inhibitor (SSRI). It typically takes about a week for clients to begin to notice the therapeutic effects of drugs in this category, and it may take several more weeks to feel these drugs' therapeutic peak.

 NCLEX® Connection: Pharmacological Therapies, Expected Actions/Outcomes

| UNIT 4 | PSYCHOPHARMACOLOGIC THERAPIES |
| Chapter 19 | Medications for Depression |

Overview

- Depression is a mood (affective) disorder that is a prevalent disease, ranking high among causes of disability.

- Advise clients starting antidepressant medication therapy for depression that symptom relief can take 1 to 3 weeks, and possibly 2 to 3 months, for full therapeutic benefits to be reached. Encourage continued compliance.

- Clients diagnosed with major depression may require hospitalization with the implementation of close observation and suicide precautions until antidepressant medications reach their peak effect.

- Antidepressant mediations are classified into four main groups:

  o Tricyclic antidepressants (TCAs)

  o Selective serotonin reuptake inhibitors (SSRIs)

  o Monoamine oxidase inhibitors (MAOIs)

  o Atypical antidepressants

MEDICATION CLASSIFICATION: TRICYCLIC ANTIDEPRESSANTS (TCAs)

- Select Prototype Medication: amitriptyline (Elavil)

- Other Medications

  o Imipramine (Tofranil)

  o Doxepin (Sinequan)

  o Nortriptyline (Aventyl)

  o Trimipramine (Surmontil)

Purpose

- Expected Pharmacological Action

  o These medications block reuptake of norepinephrine and serotonin in the synaptic space, thereby intensifying the effects of these neurotransmitters.

- Therapeutic Uses
  - Depression
  - Depressive episodes of bipolar disorders
- Other Uses
  - Chronic pain
  - Enuresis

Complications

SIDE/ADVERSE EFFECTS	NURSING INTERVENTIONS/CLIENT EDUCATION
Orthostatic hypotension	• Instruct clients about the signs of orthostatic hypotension (lightheadedness, dizziness). Advise clients to change positions slowly and to sit or lie down if symptoms occur. • Monitor the hospitalized client's blood pressure (BP) and heart rate for orthostatic changes. If a significant decrease in blood pressure or increase in heart rate is noted, do not administer the medication, and notify the provider.

Anticholinergic effects
• Dry mouth
• Blurred vision
• Photophobia
• Urinary hesitancy or retention
• Constipation
• Tachycardia
	• Instruct clients on ways to minimize anticholinergic effects. These include:
	  ○ Chewing sugarless gum
	  ○ Sipping water
	  ○ Wearing sunglasses when outdoors
	  ○ Eating foods high in fiber
	  ○ Exercising regularly
	  ○ Increasing fluid intake to at least 2 to 3 L/day from beverage and food sources
	  ○ Voiding just before taking the medication
	• Advise clients to notify the provider if symptoms persist.

Sedation	• Advise clients that this effect usually diminishes over time. • Advise clients to avoid hazardous activities (driving) if sedation is excessive. • Advise the client to take medication at bedtime to minimize daytime sleepiness and to promote sleep.
Toxicity resulting in cholinergic blockade and cardiac toxicity evidenced by dysrhythmias, mental confusion, and agitation, which are followed by seizures, coma, and possible death	• Give a 1-week supply of medication to clients who are acutely ill. • Obtain the client's baseline ECG. • Monitor vital signs frequently. • Monitor clients for signs of toxicity. • Notify the provider if signs of toxicity occur.
Decreased seizure threshold	• Monitor clients who have seizure disorders.
Excessive sweating	• Inform clients of this side effect.

(S) Contraindications/Precautions

- TCAs are Pregnancy Risk Category C.

- These medications are contraindicated for clients who have seizure disorders.

- Use cautiously in clients with coronary artery disease; diabetes; liver, kidney and respiratory disorders; urinary retention and obstruction; angle closure glaucoma; benign prostatic hypertrophy; and hyperthyroidism.

Interactions

MEDICATION/FOOD INTERACTIONS	NURSING INTERVENTIONS/ CLIENT EDUCATION
Concurrent use with MAOIs may cause hypertension, which may become severe.	Avoid concurrent use of TCAs and MAOIs.
Concurrent use with antihistamines and other anticholinergic agents may result in additive anticholinergic effects.	Avoid concurrent use of TCAs and antihistamines.
Increased effects of epinephrine and dopamine (direct-acting sympathomimetics) occur because uptake into the nerve terminals is blocked by TCAs and they remain for a longer amount of time in the synaptic space.	Avoid concurrent use of TCAs and these medications.
TCAs decrease the effects of ephedrine, amphetamine (indirect-acting sympathomimetics), because uptake into the nerve terminals is blocked and they are unable to reach their site of action.	Avoid concurrent use of TCAs and these medications.
Concurrent use with alcohol, benzodiazepines, opioids, and antihistamines may result in additive CNS depression.	Advise clients to avoid other CNS depressants.

MEDICATION CLASSIFICATION: SELECTIVE SEROTONIN REUPTAKE INHIBITORS (SSRIs)

- Select Prototype Medication: fluoxetine (Prozac)

- Other Medications

  o Citalopram (Celexa)

  o Escitalopram (Lexapro)

  o Paroxetine (Paxil)

  o Sertraline (Zoloft)

Purpose

- Expected Pharmacological Action

  o SSRIs selectively block reuptake of the monoamine neurotransmitter serotonin in the synaptic space, thereby intensifying the effects of serotonin.

- Therapeutic Uses

  o Major depression

  o Obsessive compulsive disorder (OCD)

  o Bulimia nervosa

  o Premenstrual dysphoric disorders

  o Panic disorders

  o Posttraumatic disorder (PTSD)

Complications

SIDE/ADVERSE EFFECTS	NURSING INTERVENTIONS/CLIENT EDUCATION
Sexual dysfunction (anorgasmia, impotence, decreased libido)	• Warn clients of possible side effects and to notify the provider if they become intolerable. • Instruct clients to report problems with sexual function (may be managed with dose reduction, medication holiday, changing medications).
CNS stimulation (inability to sleep, agitation, anxiety)	• Advise clients to notify the provider. Provider may decrease dosage. • Advise clients to take this medication in the morning. • Advise clients to avoid caffeinated beverages. • Instruct clients to practice relaxation techniques to promote sleep.
Occurrence of weight loss early in therapy that may be followed by weight gain with long-term treatment	• Monitor the client's weight. • Encourage clients to participate in regular exercise and to follow a healthy, well-balanced diet.
Serotonin syndrome may begin 2 to 72 hr after the start of treatment, and it may be lethal. Manifestations include mental confusion or difficulty concentrating, agitation, fever, anxiety, hallucinations, hyperreflexia or incoordination, diaphoresis, and tremors.	• Advise clients to observe for symptoms and to notify the provider immediately if they occur.
Withdrawal syndrome (headache, nausea, visual disturbances, anxiety, dizziness, tremors)	• Advise clients not to discontinue use abruptly. • Advise clients how to slowly taper the medication dosage after a long period of use to avoid withdrawal symptoms.
Hyponatremia, which is more likely to occur in older adult clients taking diuretics	• Obtain a baseline serum sodium, and monitor the level periodically throughout treatment.

SIDE/ADVERSE EFFECTS	NURSING INTERVENTIONS/CLIENT EDUCATION
Rash	• Advise clients to treat a rash with an antihistamine and to notify the provider.
Sleepiness, faintness, and lightheadedness	• Advise clients that these side effects are not common, but can occur. • Advise clients not to drive if these side effects occur.
Gastrointestinal bleeding	• Use cautiously in clients with a history of gastrointestinal (GI) bleeding, ulcers, and those taking NSAIDs or anticoagulants.

Bruxism	• Advise clients to report this to the provider who may:
	   ○ Switch clients to another class of medication.
	   ○ Treat bruxism with low-dose buspirone.
	• Advise clients to use a mouth guard during sleep.

 Contraindications/Precautions

- Fluoxetine is a Pregnancy Risk Category C medication.

- Fluoxetine and paroxetine may increase the risk of birth defects. The provider may prescribe other SSRIs. Late in pregnancy, use of SSRIs may increase the risk of withdrawal symptoms or pulmonary hypertension in the newborn.

- These medications are contraindicated in clients taking MAOIs or TCAs.

- Use cautiously in clients with liver and/or renal dysfunction, cardiac disease, seizure disorders, diabetes, ulcers, and a history of gastrointestinal bleeding and those taking NSAIDs or anticoagulants.

Interactions

MEDICATION/FOOD INTERACTIONS	NURSING INTERVENTIONS/CLIENT EDUCATION
Concurrent use with MAOIs, TCAs, and St. John's Wort increases the risk of serotonin syndrome.	• MAOIs should be discontinued for 14 days prior to starting an SSRI. Fluoxetine should be discontinued 2 to 5 weeks before starting an MAOI. • Advise clients against concurrent use of SSRIs and St. John's Wort.
Fluoxetine can displace warfarin (Coumadin) from bound protein and result in increased warfarin levels.	• Monitor the client's PT and INR levels. • Monitor clients for signs of bleeding and the need for dosage adjustment.
Fluoxetine can increase the levels of tricyclic antidepressants and lithium.	• Avoid concurrent use.
Fluoxetine suppresses platelet aggregation and thus increases the risk of bleeding when used concurrently with NSAIDs and anticoagulants.	• Advise clients to monitor for signs of bleeding (bruising, hematuria) and to notify the provider if they occur.

MEDICATION CLASSIFICATION: MONOAMINE OXIDASE INHIBITORS (MAOIs)

- Select Prototype Medication: phenelzine (Nardil)

- Other Medications

  o Isocarboxazid (Marplan)

  o Tranylcypromine (Parnate)

  o Selegiline (Emsam) – Transdermal patch

Purpose

- Expected Pharmacological Action

  o These medications block MAO-A in the brain, thereby increasing the amount of norepinephrine, dopamine, and serotonin available for transmission of impulses. An increased amount of those neurotransmitters at nerve endings intensifies responses and relieves depression.

- Therapeutic Uses

  o Atypical depression

  o Bulimia nervosa

  o OCD

  o Panic Disorder

Complications

SIDE/ADVERSE EFFECTS	NURSING INTERVENTIONS/CLIENT EDUCATION
CNS stimulation (anxiety, agitation, hypomania, mania)	• Advise clients to observe for symptoms and to notify the provider if they occur.
Orthostatic hypotension	• Monitor the client's BP and heart rate for orthostatic changes. • Hold the medication, and notify the provider regarding significant changes. • Advise clients to change positions slowly.
Hypertensive crisis (severe hypertension as a result of intensive vasoconstriction and stimulation of the heart) resulting from intake of dietary tyramine. Manifestations may include headache, nausea, increased heart rate, and increased blood pressure	• Assist with emergency care.
Local rash associated with transdermal preparation	• Instruct clients to choose a clean, dry area for each application. • Instruct clients to apply a topical glucocorticoid on the affected areas if rash occurs.

Ⓢ Contraindications/Precautions

- Phenelzine is a Pregnancy Risk Category C medication.

- MAOIs are contraindicated in clients taking SSRIs or clients with pheochromocytoma, cardiovascular and cerebral vascular disease, and/or severe renal insufficiency.

- Use cautiously in clients with diabetes and/or seizure disorders or those taking TCAs.

- Transdermal selegiline is contraindicated for clients taking carbamazepine (Tegretol) or oxcarbazepine (Trileptal). Concurrent use of these medications may increase blood levels of the MAOI.

Interactions

MEDICATION/FOOD INTERACTIONS	NURSING INTERVENTIONS/CLIENT EDUCATION
Indirect-acting sympathomimetic medications (ephedrine, amphetamine) promote the release of norepinephrine and lead to hypertensive crisis.	• Instruct clients to avoid over-the-counter decongestants and cold remedies, which frequently contain medications with sympathomimetic action.
Concurrent use with TCAs and MAOIs can lead to hypertensive crisis.	• Avoid concurrent use.
Use with SSRIs can lead to serotonin syndrome.	• Avoid concurrent use.
Concurrent use with antihypertensives may cause additive hypotensive effects.	• Monitor the client's BP. • Notify the provider if there is a significant drop in the client's BP, as the provider may reduce the dosage.
Use with meperidine (Demerol) can lead to hyperpyrexia.	• Use an alternative analgesic.
Hypertensive crisis can result from intake of dietary tyramine.	• Monitor clients for ability to follow strict adherence to dietary restrictions. • Give written information regarding tyramine-rich foods, including aged cheese, pepperoni, salami, avocados, figs, bananas, smoked fish, protein, dietary supplements, some beers, and red wine. • Advise clients to avoid taking any medications without approval from the provider. • Inform clients of symptoms and to notify the provider if they occur.
Concurrent use with vasopressors (caffeine, phenylethylamine) may result in hypertension.	• Advise clients to avoid foods that contain these agents (caffeinated beverages, chocolate, fava beans, ginseng).

MEDICATION CLASSIFICATION: ATYPICAL ANTIDEPRESSANTS

- Select Prototype Medication: bupropion HCL (Wellbutrin)

Purpose

- Expected Pharmacological Action
  - This medication acts by inhibiting dopamine uptake.
- Therapeutic Uses
  - Treatment of depression
  - Alternative to SSRIs for clients unable to tolerate the sexual dysfunction side effects
  - Aid to quit smoking
  - Prevention of seasonal affective disorder (SAD)

Complications

SIDE/ADVERSE EFFECTS	NURSING INTERVENTIONS/CLIENT EDUCATION
Headache, dry mouth, GI distress, constipation, increased heart rate, nausea, restlessness, and insomnia	• Advise clients to observe for symptoms and to notify the provider if they become intolerable. • Recommend clients treat headaches with a mild analgesic. • Advise clients to sip fluids to treat dry mouth, and to increase dietary fiber to prevent constipation.
Suppression of appetite resulting in weight loss	• Monitor the client's food intake and weight.
Seizures, especially at higher dose ranges	• Avoid use with clients at risk for seizures (head injury). • Monitor clients for seizures, and treat accordingly.

 Contraindications/Precautions

- Bupropion HCL is a Pregnancy Risk Category B medication.
- This medication should be used cautiously in clients with a seizure disorder.
- This medication is contraindicated in clients taking MAOIs.

Interactions

MEDICATION/FOOD INTERACTIONS	NURSING INTERVENTIONS/CLIENT EDUCATION
MAOIs (phenelzine [Nardil]) may increase the risk for toxicity.	• Discontinue MAOIs 2 weeks prior to beginning treatment with bupropion HCL.

OTHER ATYPICAL ANTIDEPRESSANTS

PHARMACOLOGICAL ACTION	NURSING INTERVENTIONS/CLIENT EDUCATION
Venlafaxine (Effexor) and Duloxetine (Cymbalta) (SNRIs)	
These medications inhibit serotonin and norepinephrine reuptake, thereby increasing the amount of these neurotransmitters available in the brain for impulse transmission. There is also a minimal amount of dopamine blockade.	• Inform clients that side effects include headache, nausea, agitation, anxiety, and sleep disturbances. • Monitor for hyponatremia, especially in older adult clients. • Monitor clients for weight loss. • Monitor clients for increases in diastolic blood pressure. • Discuss ways to manage interference with sexual functioning. • Advise clients to avoid abrupt cessation of the medication.
Mirtazapine (Remeron)	
This medication increases the release of serotonin and norepinephrine, thereby increasing the amount of these neurotransmitters available for impulse transmission.	• Inform clients that therapeutic effects may occur sooner, and with less sexual dysfunction, than with SSRIs. • Inform clients that this medication is generally well tolerated but they may experience weight gain, elevated cholesterol, and sleepiness that can be exacerbated by other CNS depressants.
Reboxetine (Edronax)	
This agent selectively inhibits the reuptake of norepinephrine, thereby increasing the amount of neurotransmitters available for impulse transmission.	• Inform clients that reboxetine is generally well tolerated, but clients may experience dry mouth, decreased blood pressure, constipation, sexual dysfunction, and urinary hesitancy or retention.
Trazodone (Desyrel)	
This medication has moderate selective blockade of serotonin receptors, thereby increasing the amount of that neurotransmitter available for impulse transmission.	• Inform clients that priapism may be a serious side effect, and they should seek medical attention immediately if this occurs. • Sedation may be an issue; therefore, clients taking an SSRI may benefit from its use.

Nursing Administration

- Monitor clients for suicidal thoughts during the first few weeks of therapy as the client's energy may increase without relieving symptoms, thereby placing clients at risk for suicide.

- Instruct clients to take this medication as prescribed on a daily basis to establish therapeutic plasma levels.

- Assist with the client's medication regimen adherence by informing the client that therapeutic effects may not be experienced for 1 to 3 weeks. Full therapeutic effects may take 2 to 3 months.

- Instruct clients to continue therapy after improvement in symptoms. Sudden discontinuation of the medication can result in relapse.

- Advise clients that therapy usually continues for 6 months after resolution of symptoms, and it may continue for a year or longer.

- (S) Facilitate suicide prevention by recommending the provider prescribe only a week's worth of medication for an acutely ill client, especially with TCAs.

- For SSRIs:

  o Advise clients to take these medications in the morning to minimize sleep disturbances.

  o Advise clients to take these medications with food to minimize GI disturbances.

  o (G) Obtain baseline sodium levels for older adult clients taking diuretics; monitor these clients regularly.

- For MAOIs:

  o Give clients a list of tyramine-rich foods to avoid to prevent a hypertensive crisis.

  o Advise clients to avoid taking any other prescription or nonprescription medications unless approved by the provider.

- For bupropion HCL:

  o Advise clients with Seasonal Affective Disorder to take medication beginning in the autumn each year and gradually taper dose and discontinue by spring.

Nursing Evaluation of Medication Effectiveness

- Depending on therapeutic intent, effectiveness may be evidenced by:

  o Verbalizing improvement in mood

  o Ability to perform ADLs

  o Improved sleeping and eating habits

  o Increased interaction with peers

Ⓐ **APPLICATION EXERCISES**

1. A nurse is reinforcing teaching with a client who has a new prescription for imipramine (Tofranil). Which of the following statements made by the client indicates that he understood the instructions?

    A. "I should reduce my fiber intake for a few weeks."

    B. "I may feel drowsy for a few weeks after I start taking this medicine."

    C. "I cannot eat my favorite pizza with pepperoni anymore."

    D. "I know I must take this medication until I begin to feel better."

2. A nurse is caring for a client who is taking phenelzine (Nardil). For which of the following adverse effects should the nurse monitor the client? (Select all that apply.)

    _____ Elevated blood glucose level

    _____ Nausea

    _____ Somnolence

    _____ Headache

    _____ Bruxism

3. A client has been prescribed bupropion HCL (Wellbutrin) for depression. After reviewing the client's medical record, the nurse should report which of the following findings to the client's provider immediately?

    A. The client has a family history of depression.

    B. The client swims three times a week for exercise.

    C. The client had a head injury from a motor-vehicle crash last year.

    D. The client has been dieting and lost 4.5 kg (10 lb) over the last year.

4. Which of the following antidepressants can cause the serious adverse effect of priapism?

    A. Mirtazapine (Remeron)

    B. Venlafaxine (Effexor)

    C. Trazodone (Desyrel)

    D. Imipramine (Tofranil)

5. A client has a new prescription for citalopram (Celexa).Which of the following must the nurse make sure the client is not also taking? (Select all that apply.)

    _____ A monoamine oxidase inhibitor (MAOI)

    _____ A tricyclic antidepressant (TCA)

    _____ St. John's wort

    _____ A nonsteroidal anti-inflammatory drug (NSAID)

    _____ Supplemental iron

(A) **APPLICATION EXERCISES ANSWER KEY**

1. A nurse is reinforcing teaching with a client who has a new prescription for imipramine (Tofranil). Which of the following statements made by the client indicates that he understood the instructions?

    A. "I should reduce my fiber intake for a few weeks."

    B. "I may feel drowsy for a few weeks after I start taking this medicine."

    C. "I cannot eat my favorite pizza with pepperoni anymore."

    D. "I know I must take this medication until I begin to feel better."

    Sedation is a side effect of imipramine, a tricyclic antidepressant (TCA), during the first few weeks of therapy. Usually this is self-limiting. Constipation is an adverse effect, so the client should consume a moderate amount of high-fiber foods. Clients should avoid tyramine-rich foods such as pepperoni if prescribed a monoamine oxidase inhibitor. Orthostatic hypotension is expected with TCAs.

    (N) **NCLEX® Connection: Pharmacological Therapies, Adverse Effects/Contraindications/Side Effects/Interactions**

2. A nurse is caring for a client who is taking phenelzine (Nardil). For which of the following adverse effects should the nurse monitor the client? (Select all that apply.)

    _____ Elevated blood glucose level

    __**X**__ **Nausea**

    _____ Somnolence

    __**X**__ **Headache**

    _____ Bruxism

    Nausea and headache are adverse effects of phenelzine. It does not result in elevated blood glucose levels, agitation rather than somnolence can result, and bruxism is a side effect of fluoxetine (Prozac) and not of phenelzine.

    (N) **NCLEX® Connection: Pharmacological Therapies, Adverse Effects/Contraindications/Side Effects/Interactions**

3. A client has been prescribed bupropion HCL (Wellbutrin) for depression. After reviewing the client's medical record, the nurse should report which of the following findings to the client's provider immediately?

   A. The client has a family history of depression.

   B. The client swims three times a week for exercise.

   C. The client had a head injury from a motor-vehicle crash last year.

   D. The client has been dieting and lost 4.5 kg (10 lb) over the last year.

   The greatest risk to this client is the development of seizures. Because bupropion HCL can lower the seizure threshold, clients with a history of a head injury should not take this drug. This client's family history of depression, usual activities, and current nutritional status are important but do not warrant immediate reporting to the provider.

   Ⓝ NCLEX® Connection: Pharmacological Therapies, Adverse Effects/Contraindications/Side Effects/Interactions

4. Which of the following antidepressants can cause the serious adverse effect of priapism?

   A. Mirtazapine (Remeron)

   B. Venlafaxine (Effexor)

   C. Trazodone (Desyrel)

   D. Imipramine (Tofranil)

   Trazodone can cause priapism, warranting immediate medical care. Although mirtazapine, venlafaxine, and imipramine can cause other adverse urogenital effects, they do not cause priapism.

   Ⓝ NCLEX® Connection: Pharmacological Therapies, Adverse Effects/Contraindications/Side Effects/Interactions

5. A client has a new prescription for citalopram (Celexa).Which of the following must the nurse make sure the client is not also taking? (Select all that apply.)

X	**A monoamine oxidase inhibitor (MAOI)**
X	**A tricyclic antidepressant (TCA)**
X	**St. John's wort**
____	A nonsteroidal anti-inflammatory drug (NSAID)
____	Supplemental iron

   Citalopram is a selective serotonin reuptake inhibitor (SSRI). Taking it with an SSRI, MAOIs, TCAs, and St. John's wort can increase the risk of serotonin syndrome, a serious complication. It is generally considered safe to take an SSRI with NSAIDs or with supplemental iron.

   Ⓝ NCLEX® Connection: Pharmacological Therapies, Adverse Effects/Contraindications/Side Effects/Interactions

UNIT 4	PSYCHOPHARMACOLOGIC THERAPIES
Chapter 20	Medications for Bipolar Disorders

Overview

- Medications for bipolar disorder include:

    o Mood stabilizers – lithium carbonate (Lithane, Eskalith, Lithobid)

    o Mood-stabilizing antiepileptic drugs (AEDs)

        ▪ Carbamazepine (Tegretol)

        ▪ Valproic acid (Depakote)

        ▪ Lamotrigine (Lamictal)

    o Atypical antipsychotics – These can be useful in early treatment to promote sleep and to decrease anxiety and agitation. These medications also demonstrate mood-stabilizing properties.

    o Anxiolytics – Clonazepam (Klonopin) and lorazepam (Ativan) can be useful in treating acute mania and managing the psychomotor agitation often seen in mania.

MEDICATION CLASSIFICATION: MOOD STABILIZER

- Select Prototype Medication: lithium carbonate

Purpose

- Expected Pharmacological Action

    o Lithium carbonate produces neurochemical changes in the brain, including serotonin receptor blockade.

    o There is evidence that lithium carbonate decreases neuronal atrophy and/or increases neuronal growth.

- Therapeutic Uses

    o Lithium carbonate controls episodes of acute mania, helps to prevent the return of mania or depression, and decreases the incidence of suicide.

    o Other uses include:

        ▪ Alcoholism

        ▪ Bulimia

        ▪ Schizophrenia

Complications

- Effects of therapeutic lithium carbonate levels – Some effects will resolve within a few weeks.

SIDE/ADVERSE EFFECTS	NURSING INTERVENTIONS/CLIENT EDUCATION
Gastrointestinal (GI) distress (nausea, diarrhea, abdominal pain)	• Advise clients that symptoms are usually transient. • Suggest clients take medication with meals or milk.
Fine hand tremors that can interfere with purposeful motor skills and can be exacerbated by factors such as stress and caffeine	• Use a beta$_2$-adrenergic blocking agent, such as propranolol (Inderal), to control tremors. • Administer the lowest effective dose. • Advise clients to report an increase in tremors, which could be a sign of lithium carbonate toxicity.
Polyuria and mild thirst	• Instruct clients to maintain adequate fluid intake by consuming at least 2 to 3 L of fluid/day from beverages or food sources.
Weight gain	• Assist clients to follow a healthy diet and regular exercise regimen.
Renal toxicity	• Monitor the client's I&O. • Monitor baseline BUN and creatinine, and monitor kidney function periodically.
Goiter and hypothyroidism with long-term treatment	• Obtain the client's baseline T$_3$, T$_4$, and TSH levels prior to starting treatment, and then annually. • Advise clients to monitor for signs of hypothyroidism (cold, dry skin; decreased heart rate; weight gain). • Use levothyroxine (Synthroid) to manage hypothyroidism.
Bradydysrhythmia, hypotension, and electrolyte imbalances	• Encourage clients to maintain adequate fluid intake.

- Signs and symptoms of toxicity

SIGNS AND SYMPTOMS OF TOXICITY	NURSING INTERVENTIONS/CLIENT EDUCATION
Early Signs – Less than 1.5 mEq/L	
Diarrhea, nausea, vomiting, thirst, polyuria, muscle weakness, and slurred speech	• Instruct clients to discontinue the medication, and notify the provider. • Administer new dosage if ordered based on the client's serum lithium carbonate levels.
Advanced Signs – 1.5 to 2.0 mEq/L	
Mental confusion, poor coordination, coarse tremors, and ongoing gastrointestinal distress, including nausea, vomiting, and diarrhea	• Instruct clients to discontinue the medication, and notify the provider. • Administer new dosage if ordered based on the client's serum lithium carbonate levels.

SIGNS AND SYMPTOMS OF TOXICITY	NURSING INTERVENTIONS/CLIENT EDUCATION
Severe Toxicity – 2.0 to 2.5 mEq/L	
Extreme polyuria of dilute urine, tinnitus, blurred vision, ataxia, seizures, severe hypotension leading to coma, and possible death from respiratory complications	• Administer an emetic to clients who are alert. • Assist with clients undergoing gastric lavage. • Assist with clients who are receiving medications to increase the rate of excretion.
Severe Toxicity – Greater than 2.5 mEq/L	
Rapid progression of symptoms leading to coma and death	• Hemodialysis may be warranted.

 Contraindications/Precautions

- Lithium carbonate is a Pregnancy Risk Category D medication. It is considered teratogenic, especially during the first trimester of pregnancy.

- Discuss alternatives to breastfeeding if lithium carbonate therapy is necessary.

- Use cautiously in clients with renal dysfunction, heart disease, sodium depletion, and dehydration.

Interactions

MEDICATION/FOOD INTERACTIONS	NURSING INTERVENTIONS/CLIENT EDUCATION
Diuretics – Sodium is excreted with the use of diuretics. With decreased serum sodium, lithium carbonate excretion is decreased, which can lead to toxicity.	• Monitor clients for signs of toxicity. • Advise clients to observe for symptoms and to notify the provider. • Encourage clients to maintain a diet adequate in sodium and to drink 2,000 to 3,000 mL of water/day.
NSAIDs (ibuprofen [Motrin], celecoxib [Celebrex]) – Concurrent use will increase renal reabsorption of lithium carbonate, leading to toxicity.	• Encourage clients to avoid these NSAIDs and to use aspirin as a mild analgesic.
Anticholinergics (antihistamines, tricyclic antidepressants) – Abdominal discomfort can result from anticholinergic-induced urinary retention and polyuria caused by lithium.	• Advise clients to avoid medications with anticholinergic effects.

Nursing Administration

- Monitor serum lithium carbonate levels while undergoing treatment. At initiation of treatment, monitor levels every 2 to 3 days until stable, and then every 1 to 3 months. Obtain lithium carbonate blood levels in the morning, usually 12 hr after last dose.

  - During initial treatment of a manic episode, levels should be 0.8 to 1.4 mEq/L.

  - Maintenance level range is 0.4 to 1.0 mEq/L.

  - Serum levels greater than 1.5 mEq/L can result in toxicity.

- Care for a client with a toxic serum lithium carbonate level should take place in an inpatient setting and supportive measures provided. Hemodialysis may be indicated.

- Advise clients that antimanic effects begin within 5 to 7 days and may take 2 to 3 weeks to achieve full benefits.

- Advise clients to take lithium carbonate as prescribed, usually in 2 to 3 doses daily, due to a short half-life. Taking lithium carbonate with food will help decrease GI distress.

- Encourage clients to adhere to laboratory appointments needed to monitor lithium carbonate effectiveness and adverse effects. Emphasize the high risk of toxicity due to the narrow therapeutic range.

- Provide nutritional counseling. Stress the importance of adequate fluid and sodium intake.

- Instruct clients to monitor for signs of toxicity and when to contact the provider. Clients should stop taking medication and seek medical attention if experiencing diarrhea, vomiting, or excessive sweating.

MEDICATION CLASSIFICATION: MOOD-STABILIZING ANTIEPILEPTIC DRUGS (AEDs)

- Select Prototype Medications

  - Carbamazepine (Tegretol)

  - Valproic acid (Depakote)

  - Lamotrigine (Lamictal)

Purpose

- Expected Pharmacological Action

  - AEDs help treat and manage bipolar disorder through various mechanisms, which include:

    - Slowing the entrance of sodium and calcium back into the neuron, thus extending the time it takes for the nerve to return to its active state

    - Potentiating the inhibitory effects of the neurotransmitter gamma butyric acid (GABA)

    - Inhibiting glutamic acid (glutamate), which in turn suppresses CNS excitation

- Therapeutic Uses

  o Treatment of manic and depressive episodes, relapse of mania and depressive episodes

  o Particularly useful for clients who have mixed mania and for clients who have rapid cycling bipolar disorder

Complications

SIDE/ADVERSE EFFECTS	NURSING INTERVENTIONS/CLIENT EDUCATION
Carbamazepine (Tegretol)	
• Minimal effect on cognitive function • CNS effects include nystagmus, double vision, vertigo, staggering gait, and headache	• Administer in low doses initially, and then gradually increase dosage. • Advise clients that symptoms should subside within a few weeks. • Administer dose at bedtime.
• Blood dyscrasias (leukopenia, anemia, thrombocytopenia)	• Obtain the client's baseline CBC and platelet level. Perform ongoing monitoring of these. • Observe clients for signs of bruising and bleeding of gums and instruct clients to monitor for these.
• Teratogenesis	• Advise clients to avoid use in pregnancy.
• Hypo-osmolarity – Promotes secretion of ADH, which inhibits water excretion by the kidneys, and places clients with heart failure at risk for fluid overload	• Monitor the client's serum sodium. • Monitor clients for edema, decrease in urine output, and hypertension.
• Skin disorders include dermatitis and rash (Stevens-Johnson syndrome)	• Treat mild reactions with anti-inflammatory or antihistamine medications. • Advise clients to wear sunscreen. • Instruct clients to discontinue the medication, and notify the provider if rash occurs.

SIDE/ADVERSE EFFECTS	NURSING INTERVENTIONS/CLIENT EDUCATION
Valproic Acid (Depakote)	
• GI effects include nausea, vomiting, and indigestion	• Advise clients that these symptoms are generally self-limiting. • Advise clients to take medication with food, or request an enteric-coated formulation.
• Hepatotoxicity (anorexia, nausea, vomiting, fatigue, abdominal pain, and jaundice)	• Monitor baseline liver function, and monitor liver function regularly. • Advise clients to observe for signs and symptoms of hepatotoxicity and to notify the provider immediately if they occur. • Administer the lowest effective dose.
• Pancreatitis (nausea, vomiting, and abdominal pain)	• Advise clients to observe for signs and symptoms of pancreatitis and to notify the provider immediately if they occur. • Monitor amylase levels. • Recognize that the medication will be discontinued if pancreatitis develops.
• Thrombocytopenia	• Advise clients to observe for signs and symptoms, such as bruising, and to notify the provider if these occur. • Monitor the client's platelet counts.
• Teratogenesis	• Advise clients to avoid use during pregnancy.
Lamotrigine (Lamictal)	
• Double or blurred vision, dizziness, headache, nausea, and vomiting	• Caution clients about performing activities that require concentration.
• Serious skin rashes, including Stevens-Johnson syndrome	• Instruct clients to discontinue the medication, and to notify the provider if a rash occurs.

 Contraindications/Precautions

- Carbamazepine and valproic acid are Pregnancy Risk Category D medications; lamotrigine is Pregnancy Risk Category C.

- Carbamazepine is contraindicated in clients with bone marrow suppression or with bleeding disorders.

- Valproic acid is contraindicated in clients with liver disorders.

Interactions

MEDICATION/FOOD INTERACTIONS	NURSING INTERVENTIONS/CLIENT EDUCATION
Carbamazepine (Tegretol)	
Oral contraceptives or warfarin (Coumadin) – Carbamazepine decreases the effects of these medications, due to stimulation of hepatic and drug-metabolizing enzymes.	• Advise clients to use an alternate form of birth control. • Monitor for therapeutic effects of warfarin. Administer adjusted dosages as prescribed.
Grapefruit juice – Inhibits metabolism of carbamazepine, thereby increasing blood levels of the medication.	• Advise clients to avoid drinking grapefruit juice.
Phenytoin or phenobarbital – Concurrent use decreases the effects of carbamazepine by stimulating metabolism.	• Monitor phenytoin and phenobarbital levels, and administer adjusted dosages as prescribed.
Valproic Acid (Depakote)	
Combining valproic acid with topiramate (Topamax) may cause hyperammonemia and severe CNS effects.	• Monitor ammonia levels • Advise clients to notify the provider if symptoms occur
Phenytoin or phenobarbital – Concurrent use increases the levels of these medications.	• Monitor phenytoin and phenobarbital levels, and adjust dosages as prescribed.
Lamotrigine (Lamictal)	
Carbamazepine, phenytoin, or phenobarbital – Concurrent use promotes liver drug-metabolizing enzymes, thereby decreasing the effect of lamotrigine.	• Monitor for therapeutic effects, and adjust dosages as prescribed.
Valproic acid – Concurrent use inhibits drug-metabolizing enzymes, thereby increasing the half-life of lamotrigine.	• Monitor for adverse effects, and adjust dosages as prescribed.

Nursing Evaluation of Medication Effectiveness

- Depending on therapeutic intent, effectiveness may be evidenced by:

    o Relief of acute manic symptoms (flight of ideas, obsessive talking, agitation) or depressive symptoms (fatigue, poor appetite, psychomotor retardation).

    o Verbalization of improvement in mood

    o Ability to perform ADLs

    o Improved sleeping and eating habits

    o Greater interaction with peers

Ⓐ APPLICATION EXERCISES

1. A client who has been taking lithium carbonate (Eskalith) for 6 months has recently developed symptoms of mild arthritis. He tells the nurse that he wants to start taking ibuprofen (Advil) for his pain. Which of the following is an appropriate response?

    A. "That is a good choice. Stronger analgesics would not be good for you."

    B. "Aspirin would be a better choice, because ibuprofen can raise your lithium blood level."

    C. "You will have to stop taking the lithium if you take pain medication."

    D. "Ibuprofen will make your lithium level fall too low, and your symptoms may come back."

2. Fill in the blanks:

    During initial treatment of a manic episode, lithium carbonate levels should be _____.

    Maintenance lithium carbonate level range is _____.

    Plasma levels greater than _____ can result in toxicity.

3. Which of the following medications, if given concurrently with lithium carbonate, could produce a toxic effect?

    A. Regular insulin (Humulin R)

    B. Prednisone (Deltasone)

    C. Digoxin (Lanoxin)

    D. Hydrochlorothiazide (HydroDIURIL)

4. A nurse is reinforcing teaching for a client prescribed lamotrigine (Lamictal) for bipolar disorder. Which of the following adverse effects should the nurse instruct the client to watch for and report to the provider? (Select all that apply.)

    _____ Insomnia

    _____ Blurred vision

    _____ Headache

    _____ Skin rashes

    _____ Muscle weakness

(A) APPLICATION EXERCISES ANSWER KEY

1. A client who has been taking lithium carbonate (Eskalith) for 6 months has recently developed symptoms of mild arthritis. He tells the nurse that he wants to start taking ibuprofen (Advil) for his pain. Which of the following is an appropriate response?

    A. "That is a good choice. Stronger analgesics would not be good for you."

    B. "Aspirin would be a better choice, because ibuprofen can raise your lithium blood level."

    C. "You will have to stop taking the lithium if you take pain medication."

    D. "Ibuprofen will make your lithium level fall too low, and your symptoms may come back."

    Ibuprofen is an NSAID, which increases renal lithium carbonate reabsorption; aspirin, although it is an NSAID, does not increase lithium carbonate levels. Stronger analgesics are not necessary for mild arthritis. Not all pain medications are contraindicated with the concurrent use of lithium. Ibuprofen will not make the lithium level fall too low.

    (N) NCLEX® Connection: Pharmacological Therapies, Adverse Effects/Contraindications/Side Effects/Interactions

2. Fill in the blanks:

    During initial treatment of a manic episode, lithium carbonate levels should be **between 0.8 to 1.4 mEq/L**.

    Maintenance lithium carbonate level range is **between 0.4 to 1.3 mEq/L**.

    Plasma levels greater than **1.5 mEq/L** can result in toxicity.

    (N) NCLEX® Connection: Reduction of Risk Potential, Laboratory Values

3. Which of the following medications, if given concurrently with lithium carbonate, could produce a toxic effect?

    A. Regular insulin (Humulin R)

    B. Prednisone (Deltasone)

    C. Digoxin (Lanoxin)

    D. Hydrochlorothiazide (HydroDIURIL)

    Hydrochlorothiazide is a diuretic, and can lead to decreased serum sodium. With decreased serum sodium, lithium carbonate excretion is decreased, which can lead to toxicity. Insulin, prednisone, and digoxin do not interact with lithium.

     NCLEX® Connection: Pharmacological Therapies, Adverse Effects/Contraindications/Side Effects/Interactions

4. A nurse is reinforcing teaching for a client prescribed lamotrigine (Lamictal) for bipolar disorder. Which of the following adverse effects should the nurse instruct the client to watch for and report to the provider? (Select all that apply.)

   _____ Insomnia

   __X__ **Blurred vision**

   __X__ **Headache**

   __X__ **Skin rashes**

   _____ Muscle weakness

   Blurred vision, headache, and skin rashes are common adverse effects of lamotrigine. The client is unlikely to develop insomnia or muscle weakness as a result of taking this medication.

   Ⓝ NCLEX® Connection: Pharmacological Therapies, Adverse Effects/Contraindications/Side Effects/Interactions

| UNIT 4 | PSYCHOPHARMACOLOGIC THERAPIES |
| Chapter 21 | Medications for Psychoses |

Overview

- Schizophrenia is the primary reason for the administration of antipsychotic medications.

    o The clinical course of schizophrenia usually involves acute exacerbations with intervals of semiremission.

    o Use medications to treat:

        ▪ Positive symptoms related to behavior, thought, and speech (agitation, delusions, hallucinations, tangential speech patterns)

        ▪ Negative symptoms (social withdrawal, lack of emotion, lack of energy, flattened affect, decreased motivation, decreased pleasure in activities)

    o The goals of psychopharmacological treatment for schizophrenia include:

        □ Suppression of acute episodes.

        □ Prevention of acute recurrence.

        □ Maintenance of the highest possible level of functioning.

- Conventional antipsychotic medications mainly control positive symptoms of psychosis. Use these medications for clients who are:

    o Able to take them successfully and are able to tolerate the side effects.

    o Violent or particularly aggressive.

- Atypical antipsychotic agents are medications of choice for clients receiving initial treatment, as well as for treating breakthrough episodes in clients on conventional medication therapy, as the atypical agents are more effective with fewer adverse effects.

    o Advantages of atypical antipsychotic agents include:

        ▪ Relief of both positive and negative symptoms.

        ▪ Decrease in affective symptoms (depression, anxiety) and suicidal behaviors.

        ▪ Decrease in neurocognitive symptoms (poor memory).

        ▪ Fewer or no extrapyramidal symptoms (EPS), including tardive dyskinesia, due to less dopamine blockade.

- Fewer anticholinergic effects, with the exception of clozapine (Clozaril), which has a high incidence of anticholinergic effects. This is because most of the atypical antipsychotics cause little or no blockade of cholinergic receptors.

- Less relapse.

MEDICATION CLASSIFICATION: ANTIPSYCHOTICS – CONVENTIONAL

- Select Prototype Medication: chlorpromazine (Thorazine)
- Other Medications
  - Haloperidol (Haldol), high potency
  - Fluphenazine (Prolixin), high potency
  - Molindone (Moban), medium potency
  - Loxapine (Loxitane), medium potency
  - Thioridazine (Mellaril), low potency
  - Thiothixene (Navane), high potency

Purpose

- Expected Pharmacological Action
  - The conventional antipsychotic medications block dopamine (D2), acetylcholine, histamine, and norepinephrine (NE) receptors in the brain and peripheral nervous system.
  - Inhibition of psychotic symptoms is believed to be a result of D2 blockade in the brain.
- Therapeutic Uses
  - Treatment of acute and chronic psychosis
  - Schizophrenia
  - Bipolar disorder – primarily the manic phase
  - Tourette's syndrome
  - Delusional and schizoaffective disorder
  - Dementia
  - Prevention of nausea/vomiting through blocking of dopamine in the chemoreceptor trigger zone of the medulla

Complications

SIDE/ADVERSE EFFECTS	NURSING INTERVENTIONS/CLIENT EDUCATION
Acute dystonia • Severe spasm of the tongue, neck, face, and back • Requires rapid treatment	• Monitor for side effects within a few hours (up to 5 days) after administration of first dose. • Treat these side effects with anticholinergic agents (benztropine [Cogentin], diphenhydramine [Benadryl]).
Parkinsonism • Bradykinesia • Rigidity • Shuffling gait • Drooling • Tremors	• Observe for signs and symptoms for the first month after the initiation of therapy. • Treat these side effects with benztropine, diphenhydramine, or amantadine (Symmetrel).
Akathisia • Inability to sit or stand still • Continual pacing and agitation	• Observe for signs and symptoms for the first 2 months after the initiation of treatment. • Manage symptoms with a beta$_2$-adrenergic blocker, benzodiazepines, or anticholinergic medications.

Late extrapyramidal side effects
• Tardive dyskinesia
  ○ Involuntary movements of the tongue and face (lip smacking)
  ○ Involuntary movements of the arms, legs, and trunk
	• Recognize that manifestations may occur months to years after the start of therapy, and may improve following medication change or may be permanent.
	• Administer the lowest dosage possible to control symptoms.
	• Evaluate clients after 12 months of therapy and then every 3 months. Manifestations may occur months to years after the initiation of therapy. If signs of TD appear, the provider will decrease the dosage or prescribe a different medication.
	• Use the Abnormal Involuntary Movement Scale (AIMS) to screen for the presence of EPS.

Neuroleptic malignant syndrome • Sudden high fever • Blood pressure fluctuations • Dysrhythmias • Muscle rigidity • Changes in level of consciousness • Coma	• Stop antipsychotic medication. • Assist with transfer to medical unit for cooling measures, administration of dantrolene (Dantrium) and bromocriptine (Parlodel), maintenance of hydration, and treatment of dysrhythmias. • Administer atypical agent as prescribed.

SIDE/ADVERSE EFFECTS	NURSING INTERVENTIONS/CLIENT EDUCATION

Anticholinergic effects
• Dry mouth
• Blurred vision
• Photophobia
• Urinary hesitancy or retention
• Constipation
• Tachycardia
	• Suggest the following strategies to decrease anticholinergic effects:
	   ○ Chewing sugarless gum
	   ○ Sipping on water
	   ○ Avoiding hazardous activities
	   ○ Wearing sunglasses when outdoors
	   ○ Eating foods high in fiber
	   ○ Participating in regular exercise
	   ○ Maintaining fluid intake of 2 to 3 L/day from beverages and food sources
	   ○ Voiding just before taking medication

Orthostatic hypotension	• Inform clients that this should stabilize in 2 to 3 months. • Monitor the client's blood pressure and heart rate for orthostatic changes. Hold medication until the provider is notified of significant changes. • Instruct clients about the signs of orthostatic hypotension (lightheadedness, dizziness). Instruct clients to change positions slowly and to sit or lie down if symptoms occur.
Sedation	• Inform clients that effects should diminish within a few weeks. • Instruct clients to take the medication at bedtime to avoid daytime sleepiness. • Advise clients not to drive until sedation has subsided.
Neuroendocrine effects • Gynecomastia • Galactorrhea • Menstrual irregularities	• Advise clients to observe for these manifestations and to notify the provider if they occur.
Seizures • Risk is greatest in those clients who have an existing seizure disorder.	• Advise clients to report seizure activity to the provider. • Inform clients with a seizure disorder that an increase in antiseizure medication may be necessary.
Sexual dysfunction • Common in both males and females	• Advise clients of possible side effects. • Encourage clients to report side effects to the provider. The provider may decrease the dosage or prescribe a different medication.
Skin effects • Photosensitivity that can result in severe sunburn • Contact dermatitis from handling medications	• Advise clients to avoid excessive exposure to sunlight, to use sunscreen, and to wear protective clothing. • Advise clients to avoid direct contact with the medication.

SIDE/ADVERSE EFFECTS	NURSING INTERVENTIONS/CLIENT EDUCATION
Agranulocytosis	• Advise clients to observe for signs of infection (fever, sore throat) and to notify the provider immediately if these occur. • If signs of infection appear, obtain the client's baseline WBC count. Expect the provider to discontinue the medication if infection is present.
Prolongation of QT interval leading to a fatal dysrhythmia, with chlorpromazine, or haloperidol	• Obtain the client's baseline ECG and potassium and magnesium levels prior to treatment and periodically throughout the treatment period. • Assist with maintaining serum potassium and magnesium levels within expected reference range.

 Contraindications/Precautions

- These medications are contraindicated in clients who are in a coma or those who have severe depression, Parkinson's disease, prolactin-dependent cancer of the breast, and severe hypotension.

- Use of conventional antipsychotic medications is contraindicated in older adult clients with dementia.

- Use cautiously in clients with glaucoma, paralytic ileus, prostate enlargement, heart disorders, liver or kidney disease, and seizure disorders.

Interactions

MEDICATION/FOOD INTERACTIONS	NURSING INTERVENTIONS/CLIENT EDUCATION
Anticholinergic agents – Concurrent use with these medications will increase anticholinergic effects.	• Advise clients to avoid OTC medications that contain anticholinergic agents (sleep aids).
CNS depressants – Additive CNS depressant effects with concurrent use of alcohol, opioids, and antihistamines.	• Advise clients to avoid alcohol and other medications that cause CNS depression. • Advise clients to avoid hazardous activities (driving).
Levodopa – By activating dopamine receptors, levodopa counteracts effects of antipsychotic agents.	• Avoid concurrent use of levodopa and other direct dopamine receptor agonists.
Tricyclic antidepressants, amiodarone, erythromycin prolong QT and can further prolong QT interval with chlorpromazine or haloperidol	• Avoid concurrent use with other medications that prolong QT interval.

Nursing Administration

- Monitor client to differentiate between EPS and worsening of a psychotic disorder.

- Administer anticholinergics, beta$_2$-adrenergic blockers, and benzodiazepines to control early EPS. If symptoms are intolerable, the provider may prescribe a low-potency or an atypical antipsychotic agent.

- Advise clients that antipsychotic medications do not cause addiction.

- Advise clients to take medication as prescribed and to take it on a regular schedule.

- Advise clients that some therapeutic effects may be noticeable within a few days, but significant improvement may take 2 to 4 weeks, and possibly several months for full effects.

- Consider depot preparations, administered IM once every 2 to 4 weeks, for clients with difficulty maintaining medication regimen. Inform clients that lower doses can be used with depot preparations, which will decrease the risk of adverse effects and the development of tardive dyskinesia.

- Begin administration with twice daily dosing, but switch to daily dosing at bedtime to decrease daytime drowsiness and promote sleep.

MEDICATION CLASSIFICATION: ANTIPSYCHOTICS – ATYPICAL

- Select Prototype Medication: risperidone (Risperdal)

- Other Medications

  - Olanzapine (Zyprexa)

  - Quetiapine (Seroquel)

  - Aripiprazole (Abilify)

  - Ziprasidone (Geodon)

  - Clozapine (Clozaril)

Purpose

- Expected Pharmacological Action

  - These antipsychotic agents work mainly by blocking serotonin, and to a lesser degree, dopamine receptors.

  - These medications also block receptors for norepinephrine, histamine, and acetylcholine.

- Therapeutic Uses

  - Negative and positive symptoms of schizophrenia

  - Psychosis induced by levodopa therapy

  - Relief of psychotic symptoms in other disorders (bipolar disorder)

Complications

SIDE/ADVERSE EFFECTS	NURSING INTERVENTIONS/CLIENT EDUCATION
New onset of diabetes mellitus or loss of glucose control in clients with diabetes	• Obtain the client's baseline fasting blood glucose level, and monitor regularly throughout treatment. • Instruct clients to report symptoms, such as increased thirst, urination, and appetite, to the provider.
Weight gain	• Advise clients to follow a healthy, low-caloric diet, engage in regular exercise, and monitor weight gain.
Hypercholesterolemia with increased risk for hypertension and other cardiovascular disease	• Monitor the client's cholesterol, triglycerides, and blood glucose level if weight gain is greater than 14 kg (30 lb).
Orthostatic hypotension	• Monitor the client's blood pressure and heart rate for orthostatic changes. • Hold medication while notifying the provider of significant changes.
Anticholinergic effects – Urinary hesitancy, retention; dry mouth	• Monitor for these adverse effects, and report their occurrence to the provider. • Encourage clients to use measures to relieve dry mouth (sipping fluids throughout the day).
Symptoms of agitation, dizziness, sedation, and sleep disruption	• Monitor for these adverse effects, and report their occurrence to the provider. • Administer an alternative medication if prescribed.
May cause mild EPS (tremor)	• Monitor for and teach clients to recognize EPS. • Use AIMS test to screen for EPS.

Ⓢ Contraindications/Precautions

- Risperidone

    ○ Risperidone is a Pregnancy Risk Category C medication.

    ○ These medications should not be used for dementia-related psychosis. Use of these medications may cause death related to cerebrovascular accident or infection.

    ○ Clients should avoid the concurrent use of alcohol.

    ○ Use cautiously in clients with cardiovascular or cerebrovascular disease, seizures, or diabetes mellitus. Clients with diabetes mellitus should have a baseline fasting blood glucose level, and blood glucose level should be monitored carefully.

- Other Atypical Antipsychotic Agents

MEDICATION	FORMULATIONS	COMMENTS

Olanzapine (Zyprexa)	• Tablets
	• Oral solution
	• Short-acting injectable
		• Low risk of EPS
		• High risk of diabetes, weight gain, and dyslipidemia
		• Other adverse effects include:
		  ○ Sedation
		  ○ Orthostatic hypotension
		  ○ Anticholinergic effects

Quetiapine (Seroquel)	• Tablets	• Low risk of EPS
		• Moderate risk of diabetes, weight gain, and dyslipidemia
		• Other adverse effects include:
		  ○ Cataracts
		  ○ Sedation
		  ○ Orthostatic hypotension
		  ○ Anticholinergic effects

Aripiprazole (Abilify)	• Tablets
	• Oral solution
		• Low or no risk of EPS
		• Low or no risk of diabetes, weight gain, dyslipidemia, orthostatic hypotension, and anticholinergic effects
		• Adverse effects include:
		  ○ Sedation
		  ○ Headache
		  ○ Anxiety
		  ○ Insomnia
		  ○ Gastrointestinal upset

Ziprasidone (Geodon) – This medication affects both dopamine and serotonin; use for clients with concurrent depression.	• Capsules
	• Short-acting injectable
		• Low risk of EPS
		• Low risk of diabetes, weight gain, and dyslipidemia
		• Other adverse effects include:
		  ○ Sedation
		  ○ Orthostatic hypotension
		  ○ Anticholinergic effects
		  ○ ECG changes and QT prolongation that may lead to torsades de pointes

MEDICATION	FORMULATIONS	COMMENTS

Clozapine (Clozaril) – The first atypical antipsychotic developed. It is no longer considered a first-line medication for schizophrenia due to its adverse effects.	• Tablets	• Low risk of EPS
		• High risk of weight gain, diabetes, and dyslipidemia
		• Risk for fatal agranulocytosis
		   ○ Baseline and weekly monitoring of WBC recommended
		   ○ Notification of the provider of signs of infection (fever, sore throat, mouth lesions) is necessary
		• Other adverse effects include:
		   ○ Sedation
		   ○ Orthostatic hypotension
		   ○ Anticholinergic effects

(M) View Media Supplement: Reinforcing Client Education with Antipsychotic Medications (Video)

Interactions

MEDICATION/FOOD INTERACTIONS	NURSING INTERVENTIONS/CLIENT EDUCATION
Immunosuppressive medications (anticancer medications) can further suppress immune function.	• Avoid use in clients who are taking clozapine.
Additive CNS depressant effects can occur with concurrent use of alcohol, opioids, antihistamines, and other CNS depressants.	• Advise clients to avoid alcohol and other medications that cause CNS depression. • Advise clients to avoid hazardous activities (driving).
Levodopa counteracts the effects of antipsychotic agents by activating dopamine receptors.	• Avoid concurrent use of levodopa and other direct dopamine receptor agonists.
Tricyclic antidepressants, amiodarone (Cordarone), and clarithromycin (Biaxin) prolong QT intervals, thereby increasing the risk of cardiac dysrhythmias.	• Use is contraindicated with ziprasidone.
Barbiturates and phenytoin (Dilantin) stimulate hepatic drug-metabolizing enzymes, thereby decreasing drug levels of aripiprazole, quetiapine, and ziprasidone.	• Monitor medication effectiveness.
Fluconazole (Diflucan) inhibits hepatic drug-metabolizing enzymes, thereby increasing drug levels of aripiprazole, quetiapine, and ziprasidone.	• Monitor medication effectiveness.

Nursing Administration

- Administer by oral or IM route. Risperidone is also available as a depot injection administered IM once every 2 weeks. This method of administration is a good option for clients who have difficulty adhering to a medication schedule. Therapeutic effect occurs 4 to 6 weeks after first depot injection.

- Advise clients that low doses of medication are given initially and are then gradually increased.

- Use oral disintegrating tablets for clients who may attempt to "cheek" or "pocket" tablets, or for those who have difficulty swallowing them.

Nursing Evaluation of Medication Effectiveness

- Depending on therapeutic intent, effectiveness may be evidenced by:

  ○ Improvement of symptoms (prevention of acute psychotic symptoms, absence of hallucinations, delusions, anxiety, hostility)

  ○ Improvement in ability to perform ADLs

  ○ Improvement in ability to interact socially with peers

  ○ Improvement of sleeping and eating habits

Ⓐ APPLICATION EXERCISES

Scenario: A 24-year-old client with paranoid schizophrenia has been treated successfully on an outpatient basis for the past 3 years. Now his condition is deteriorating, and his provider has recommended inpatient treatment at an acute-care mental health facility. The client is suspicious of the nursing staff, and has auditory hallucinations with a voice telling him to "hurt those evil people before they hurt you." He also has pressured speech and uses clang associations. His appearance indicates a lack of grooming and hygiene. His behavior is usually aggressive toward others, but his face shows no emotion even though he sounds angry. The provider has prescribed risperidone (Risperdal) 4 mg PO once daily.

1. Which of the client's symptoms indicates a need for an atypical antipsychotic agent rather than a conventional (typical) medication?

2. What measures might the nurse suggest to the provider to enhance the effectiveness of the client's medication therapy?

3. Which of the following are common adverse effects of conventional antipsychotics such as haloperidol (Haldol)? (Select all that apply.)

    _____ Double vision

    _____ Photosensitivity

    _____ Orthostatic hypotension

    _____ Bradycardia

    _____ Seizures

4. Which of the following types of extrapyramidal effects resulting from conventional antipsychotic medications are generally the first to appear?

    A. Parkinsonism

    B. Acute dystonia

    C. Akathisia

    D. Tardive dyskinesia

5. Match the adverse effects of chlorpromazine (Thorazine) in column A with its description in column B.

    _____ Acute dystonia   A. Inability to sit still, pacing, foot tapping

    _____ Parkinsonism   B. Severe spasms of tongue, neck, face, or back

    _____ Akathisia   C. Protruding tongue, lip-smacking movements, involuntary twisting movements of the body

    _____ Tardive dyskinesia   D. Bradykinesia, rigidity, shuffling gait, drooling and tremors

(A) **APPLICATION EXERCISES ANSWER KEY**

> **Scenario:** A 24-year-old client with paranoid schizophrenia has been treated successfully on an outpatient basis for the past 3 years. Now his condition is deteriorating, and his provider has recommended inpatient treatment at an acute-care mental health facility. The client is suspicious of the nursing staff, and has auditory hallucinations with a voice telling him to "hurt those evil people before they hurt you." He also has pressured speech and uses clang associations. His appearance indicates a lack of grooming and hygiene. His behavior is usually aggressive toward others, but his face shows no emotion even though he sounds angry. The provider has prescribed risperidone (Risperdal) 4 mg PO once daily.

1. Which of the client's symptoms indicates a need for an atypical antipsychotic agent rather than a conventional (typical) medication?

    The negative symptoms of psychosis are more readily treated with atypical antipsychotics, such as risperidone, than by typical antipsychotics, such as chlorpromazine (Thorazine). Negative symptoms for the client include the lack of grooming and hygiene, and his flat affect (no facial emotion shown). His other manifestations are positive symptoms of psychosis.

(N) **NCLEX® Connection: Pharmacological Therapies, Expected Actions/Outcomes**

2. What measures might the nurse suggest to the provider to enhance the effectiveness of the client's medication therapy?

    A client who is suspicious of others and is unable to behave rationally is at a high risk for nonadherence to his treatment regimen. Risperidone is also available in orally disintegrating tablets that dissolve easily in the mouth and should keep him from "cheeking" his medication and later disposing of it. Another alternative is to administer the client's medication intramuscularly until he is able to take it orally.

(N) **NCLEX® Connection: Pharmacological Therapies, Medication Administration**

3. Which of the following are common adverse effects of conventional antipsychotics such as haloperidol (Haldol)? (Select all that apply.)

_____ Double vision

__X__ **Photosensitivity**

__X__ **Orthostatic hypotension**

_____ Bradycardia

__X__ **Seizures**

Photosensitivity, orthostatic hypotension, and seizures are common adverse effects of conventional antipsychotics. Double vision, bradycardia, and cataracts are unlikely effects of this type of medication.

(N) NCLEX® Connection: Pharmacological Therapies, Adverse Effects/Contraindications/Side Effects/Interactions

4. Which of the following types of extrapyramidal effects resulting from conventional antipsychotic medications are generally the first to appear?

A. Parkinsonism

B. Acute dystonia

C. Akathisia

D. Tardive dyskinesia

Acute dystonia generally appears anywhere between 5 hr to 5 days after the first dose. Parkinsonism appears between 5 days and 1 month. Akathisia appears between 5 days and 2 months. Tardive dyskinesia takes months to years to develop.

(N) NCLEX® Connection: Pharmacological Therapies, Adverse Effects/Contraindications/Side Effects/Interactions

5. Match the adverse effects of chlorpromazine (Thorazine) in column A with its description in column B.

__B__	Acute dystonia	A. Inability to sit still, pacing, foot tapping
__D__	Parkinsonism	B. Severe spasms of tongue, neck, face, or back
__A__	Akathisia	C. Protruding tongue, lip-smacking movements, involuntary twisting movements of the body
__C__	Tardive dyskinesia	D. Bradykinesia, rigidity, shuffling gait, drooling and tremors

(N) NCLEX® Connection: Pharmacological Therapies, Adverse Effects/Contraindications/Side Effects/Interactions

UNIT 4	PSYCHOPHARMACOLOGIC THERAPIES
Chapter 22	Medications for Children and Adolescents with Mental Health Issues

ⓐ Overview

- Use various medications to manage behavioral disorders in children and adolescents. Reinforce to parents that pharmacological management should be accompanied by behavioral modification techniques.

- Medications include SSRIs, tricyclic antidepressants, antipsychotics, nonbarbiturate anxiolytics, CNS stimulants, and norepinephrine selective reuptake inhibitors.

MEDICATION CLASSIFICATION: SSRIs

- Select Prototype Medication – fluoxetine (Prozac)

- Other Medications

  ○ Citalopram (Celexa)

  ○ Escitalopram (Lexapro)

  ○ Paroxetine (Paxil)

  ○ Sertraline (Zoloft)

Purpose

- Expected Pharmacological Action

  ○ SSRIs selectively block reuptake of the monoamine neurotransmitter serotonin in the synaptic space, thereby intensifying the effects of the serotonin.

- Therapeutic Uses

  ○ Major depression

  ○ Bulimia nervosa

  ○ Panic, school phobia, and separation anxiety disorder

  ○ Posttraumatic stress disorder (PTSD)

  ○ Obsessive compulsive disorder (OCD)

  ○ ADHD

Complications

SIDE/ADVERSE EFFECTS	NURSING INTERVENTIONS/CLIENT EDUCATION
CNS stimulation (inability to sleep, agitation, anxiety)	• Advise clients and families to notify the provider, as dose may need to be lowered. • Advise clients to take dose in the morning. • Advise clients to avoid chocolate and caffeinated beverages. • Suggest relaxation exercises to promote sleep.
Weight loss early in therapy may be followed by weight gain with long-term treatment.	• Monitor the client's weight. • Encourage clients to participate in regular exercise and to follow a healthy, well-balanced diet. • Assist clients with maintaining appropriate weight.
Serotonin syndrome may begin 2 to 72 hr after starting treatment, and it may be lethal. Manifestations include: • Mental confusion and difficulty concentrating. • Agitation. • Anxiety. • Hallucinations. • Incoordination and hyperreflexia. • Tremors. • Diaphoresis. • Fever.	• Advise clients and families to observe for symptoms and to instruct them to notify the provider immediately and stop the medication.
Withdrawal syndrome (headache, nausea, visual disturbances, anxiety)	• Reinforce to clients and families how to slowly taper the medication dosage after a long period of use to avoid withdrawal symptoms.
Rash	• Advise clients and families to treat a rash with an antihistamine and to notify the provider.
Sleepiness, faintness, and lightheadedness	• Advise clients that these side effects are not common, but they can occur.
Gastrointestinal (GI) bleeding	• Use caution in clients with a history of GI bleed and ulcers, and in clients taking other medications that affect blood coagulation.

Bruxism	• Advise clients to report to the provider, who may:
	  ○ Switch clients to another class of medication.
	  ○ Treat bruxism with low-dose buspirone.
	• Advise clients to use a mouth guard during sleep.

(S) Contraindications/Precautions

- SSRIs are contraindicated in clients taking MAOIs and tricyclic antidepressants (TCAs).

- Use cautiously in clients with liver and renal dysfunction, cardiac disease, seizure disorders, diabetes mellitus, ulcers, and a history of GI bleeding.

Interactions

MEDICATION/FOOD INTERACTIONS	NURSING INTERVENTIONS/CLIENT EDUCATION
MAOIs and TCAs – Concurrent use increases the risk of serotonin syndrome.	• Avoid concurrent use.
Warfarin (Coumadin) – Fluoxetine can displace warfarin from bound protein and result in increased warfarin levels.	• Monitor the client's PT and INR levels. • Check clients for signs of bleeding and administer new dosage as prescribed.
TCAs and lithium – Fluoxetine can increase the levels of these medications.	• Avoid concurrent use.
NSAIDs and anticoagulants – Fluoxetine suppresses platelet aggregation and thus, increases the risk of bleeding when used concurrently with these medications.	• Advise clients and families to monitor for signs of bleeding (bruising, hematuria) and to notify the provider if they occur.

Nursing Administration

- Check for the use of alcohol and other CNS depressants, especially with adolescents.

- Instruct clients to take medications with food to decrease GI distress.

- Encourage clients and families to administer the medication in the morning to minimize sleep disturbances.

- Instruct clients and families to administer the medication on a daily basis to establish therapeutic plasma levels.

- Suggest weekly dosing for clients with difficulty maintaining adherence.

- Assist clients with medication regimen compliance by informing them that optimal therapeutic effects may not be experienced for 1 to 3 weeks.

- Instruct clients and families to continue therapy after improvement in symptoms. Sudden discontinuation of medication can result in relapse.

Nursing Evaluation of Medication Effectiveness

- Effectiveness for clients diagnosed with depression may be evidenced by:

  ○ Verbalization of improvement in mood.

  ○ Improved sleeping and eating habits.

  ○ Increased interaction with peers.

- Effectiveness for clients diagnosed with ADHD may be evidenced by:

  ▪ Decreased hyperactivity.

  ▪ Increased level of concentration.

MEDICATION CLASSIFICATION: TRICYCLIC ANTIDEPRESSANTS (TCAs)

- Select Prototype Medication – Amitriptyline (Elavil)

- Other Medications:

  ○ Imipramine (Tofranil)

  ○ Clomipramine (Anafranil)

  ○ Nortriptyline (Aventyl)

Purpose

- Expected Pharmacological Action

  ○ These medications block reuptake of the monoamine neurotransmitters, norepinephrine, and serotonin in the synaptic space, thereby intensifying their effects.

- Therapeutic Uses

  ○ Depression

  ○ Depressive episodes of bipolar disorders

  ○ Autistic disorder

  ○ ADHD in children and adults

  ○ Panic, school phobia, and separation anxiety disorder

  ○ PTSD

  ○ OCD

Complications

SIDE/ADVERSE EFFECTS	NURSING INTERVENTIONS/CLIENT EDUCATION
Orthostatic hypotension	<ul><li>Monitor the client's blood pressure with the first dose.</li><li>If orthostatic hypotension occurs, instruct clients to change positions slowly.</li></ul>
Anticholinergic effects<ul><li>Dry mouth</li><li>Blurred vision</li><li>Photophobia</li><li>Urinary hesitancy or retention</li><li>Constipation</li><li>Tachycardia</li></ul>	<ul><li>Instruct clients and families regarding ways to minimize anticholinergic effects.<ul><li>Chewing sugarless gum</li><li>Sipping water</li><li>Avoiding hazardous activities</li><li>Wearing sunglasses when outdoors</li><li>Eating foods high in fiber</li><li>Participating in regular exercise</li><li>Increasing fluid intake to at least 2 to 3 L/day from beverages and other food sources</li><li>Voiding just before taking the medication</li></ul></li><li>Advise clients and families to notify the provider if symptoms become intolerable.</li></ul>
Weight gain	<ul><li>Monitor the client's weight.</li><li>Encourage clients to participate in regular exercise and to follow a healthy, low-calorie diet.</li></ul>
Sedation	<ul><li>Advise clients that side effects should diminish over time.</li><li>Advise clients to avoid hazardous activities (driving) if sedation is excessive.</li><li>Advise clients and families to administer the medication at bedtime to minimize daytime sleepiness and to promote sleep.</li></ul>
Toxicity resulting in cholinergic blockade and cardiac toxicity evidenced by dysrhythmias, mental confusion, and agitation, followed by seizures and coma	<ul><li>Give clients who are acutely ill a 1-week supply of medication.</li><li>Obtain the client's baseline ECG.</li><li>Monitor the client's vital signs frequently.</li><li>Monitor clients for signs of toxicity.</li><li>Notify the provider if signs of toxicity occur.</li></ul>
Decreased seizure threshold	<ul><li>Monitor clients with seizure disorders.</li></ul>
Excessive sweating	<ul><li>Inform clients of this side effect.</li></ul>

 Contraindications/Precautions

- Use cautiously in clients with seizure disorders; diabetes mellitus; liver, kidney and respiratory disorders; and hyperthyroidism.

Interactions

MEDICATION/FOOD INTERACTIONS	NURSING INTERVENTIONS/ CLIENT EDUCATION
MAOIs – Concurrent use may cause hypertension.	Avoid concurrent use.
Antihistamines and other anticholinergic agents – Concurrent use may cause additive anticholinergic effects.	Avoid concurrent use.
Alcohol, benzodiazepines, opioids, and antihistamines – Concurrent use may cause additive CNS depression.	Avoid concurrent use.

Nursing Administration

- Instruct clients and families to administer the medication as prescribed on a daily basis to establish therapeutic serum levels.

- Assist with the client's medication regimen adherence by informing the client that therapeutic effects may not be experienced for 1 to 3 weeks. Full therapeutic effects may not be experienced for 2 to 3 months.

- Instruct clients and families to continue therapy after improvement in symptoms. Sudden discontinuation of the medication can result in relapse.

Nursing Evaluation of Medication Effectiveness

- Effectiveness for clients diagnosed with depression may be evidenced by:
  - Verbalization of improvement in mood.
  - Improved sleeping and eating habits.
  - Increased interaction with peers.
- Effectiveness for clients diagnosed with autistic disorder may be evidenced by:
  - Decreased anger.
  - Decreased compulsive behavior.
- Effectiveness for clients diagnosed with ADHD may be evidenced by:
  - Decreased hyperactivity.
  - Increased level of concentration.

MEDICATION CLASSIFICATION: ATYPICAL ANXIOLYTIC: NONBARBITURATE ANXIOLYTIC

- Select Prototype Medication – buspirone (BuSpar)

Purpose

- Expected Pharmacological Action

  o The exact antianxiety mechanism of this medication is unknown. This medication does bind to serotonin and dopamine receptors. There is no potential for abuse, and use of buspirone does not result in sedation.

- Therapeutic Uses

  o Panic disorder

  o OCD

  o Social anxiety disorder

  o PTSD

Complications

SIDE/ADVERSE EFFECTS	NURSING INTERVENTIONS/CLIENT EDUCATION
CNS effects (dizziness, nausea, headache, agitation)	• Advise clients to take with food to decrease nausea. • Instruct clients that most side effects are self-limiting.

 Contraindications/Precautions

- Buspirone is contraindicated for concurrent use with MAOIs, or for 14 days after MAOIs are discontinued. Hypertensive crisis may result.

Interactions

MEDICATION/FOOD INTERACTIONS	NURSING INTERVENTIONS/CLIENT EDUCATION
Erythromycin, ketoconazole, and grapefruit juice increase the effect of buspirone.	• Take a complete medication history. • Advise clients to avoid drinking grapefruit juice.

Nursing Administration

- Advise clients to take the medication with meals to prevent gastric irritation.

- Advise clients and families that effects do not occur rapidly and can take a week before therapeutic benefits are felt, and several weeks before the full therapeutic benefit is felt. Advise clients and families to administer the medication on a regular basis and not PRN.

Nursing Evaluation of Medication Effectiveness

- Effectiveness for clients diagnosed with depression may be evidenced by:

  - Verbalization of improvement in mood.

  - Improved sleeping and eating habits.

  - Increased interaction with peers.

- Effectiveness for clients diagnosed with anxiety disorders may be evidenced by:

  - Decrease in anxiety symptoms.

  - Improvement in functioning.

MEDICATION CLASSIFICATION: CNS STIMULANTS

MEDICATION	SHORT ACTING	INTERMEDIATE ACTING	LONG ACTING
Methylphenidate	Ritalin, Methylin	Ritalin SR, Methylin ER	Ritalin LA, Concerta, Daytrana (transdermal)
Dexmethylphenidate	Focalin		
Dextroamphetamine	DextroStat		Dexedrine Spansules
Amphetamine mixture	Adderall		Adderall-XR

Purpose

- Expected Pharmacological Action

  - These medications raise the levels of norepinephrine, serotonin, and dopamine into the CNS.

- Therapeutic Uses

  - ADHD in children and adults

  - Conduct disorder

Complications

SIDE/ADVERSE EFFECTS	NURSING INTERVENTIONS/CLIENT EDUCATION
CNS stimulation (insomnia, restlessness)	- Advise clients and families to observe for symptoms, and if symptoms occur, instruct clients to notify the provider. - Administer the last dose of the day before 4 p.m.

SIDE/ADVERSE EFFECTS	NURSING INTERVENTIONS/CLIENT EDUCATION
Weight loss, possible growth suppression	• Monitor the client's height and weight and compare to baseline. • Administer medication immediately before, with, or right after meals. • Encourage children and adolescents to eat at regular meal times and to avoid unhealthy food choices.
Cardiovascular effects (dysrhythmias, chest pain, high blood pressure) – May increase the risk of sudden death in clients with heart abnormalities	• Monitor the client's vital signs and ECG. • Advise clients and families to observe for symptoms and to notify the provider if they occur.
Development of psychotic symptoms (hallucinations, paranoia)	• Instruct clients and families to report symptoms immediately and discontinue the medication.
Withdrawal reaction	• Advise clients to avoid abrupt cessation of the medication, as it could lead to depression and severe fatigue.
Hypersensitivity skin reaction to transdermal methylphenidate (hives, papules)	• Advise clients to remove the patch and notify the provider.

 Contraindications/Precautions

- Contraindicated in clients with a history of drug abuse, cardiovascular disorders, severe anxiety, and psychosis.

Interactions

MEDICATION/FOOD INTERACTIONS	NURSING INTERVENTIONS/CLIENT EDUCATION
MAOIs – Concurrent use may cause hypertensive crisis.	• Avoid concurrent use.
Caffeine – Concurrent use may cause an increase in CNS stimulant effects.	• Instruct clients to avoid foods and beverages that contain caffeine.
Phenytoin (Dilantin), warfarin (Coumadin), and phenobarbital – Methylphenidate inhibits metabolism of these medications leading to increased serum levels.	• Monitor clients for adverse effects (CNS depression, signs of bleeding). • Concurrent use of these medications should be used cautiously.
Over-the-counter (OTC) cold and decongestant medications – Concurrent use may lead to increased CNS stimulation.	• Instruct clients and families to avoid the use of these OTC medications.

Nursing Administration

- Advise clients to swallow sustained-release tablets whole and to not chew or crush them.

- Reinforce to clients and families the importance of administering the medication on a regular schedule.

- Reinforce to clients who use transdermal medication (Daytrana) to place the patch on one hip daily in the morning, and leave it in place no longer than 9 hr. Alternate hips daily.

- Instruct clients and families that ADHD is not cured by the medication and that an overall treatment plan should include family and cognitive therapy.

- Instruct families that these medications have special handling procedures controlled by federal law. Medication refills require handwritten prescriptions.

- Instruct families regarding safety and storage of medications.

- Advise clients and families that these medications have a high potential for abuse.

Nursing Evaluation of Medication Effectiveness

- Depending on therapeutic intent, effectiveness may be evidenced by:

  o Improvement of symptoms of ADHD, such as an increased ability to focus and complete tasks, interact with peers, and manage impulsivity.

MEDICATION CLASSIFICATION: NOREPINEPHRINE SELECTIVE REUPTAKE INHIBITOR

- Select Prototype Medication – Atomoxetine (Strattera)

Purpose

- Expected Pharmacological Action

  o Blocks reuptake of norepinephrine at synapses in the CNS. Atomoxetine is not a stimulant medication.

- Therapeutic Uses

  o ADHD in children and adults

Complications

SIDE/ADVERSE EFFECTS	NURSING INTERVENTIONS/CLIENT EDUCATION
Usually tolerated well with minimal side effects	
Appetite suppression, weight loss, and growth suppression	• Monitor the client's height and weight and compare to baseline. • Administer medication immediately before, with, or right after meals. • Encourage children and adolescents to eat at regular meal times and avoid unhealthy food choices.

SIDE/ADVERSE EFFECTS	NURSING INTERVENTIONS/CLIENT EDUCATION
Usually tolerated well with minimal side effects	
GI effects (nausea, vomiting)	• Advise clients to take the medication with food if GI effects occur.
Suicidal ideation (in children, adolescents)	• Monitor clients for signs of depression. • Advise clients and families to report changes in mood, excessive sleeping, agitation, and irritability to the provider.
Hepatotoxicity	• Advise clients to report signs of liver damage (flu-like symptoms, yellowing skin, abdominal pain).

Ⓢ Contraindications/Precautions

- Use cautiously in clients with cardiovascular disorders.

Interactions

MEDICATION/FOOD INTERACTIONS	NURSING INTERVENTIONS/CLIENT EDUCATION
MAOIs – Concurrent use may cause hypertensive crisis.	• Avoid concurrent use or within 2 weeks of each other.
Paroxetine (Paxil), fluoxetine (Prozac), or quinidine gluconate (Quinaglute Dura-Tabs) – These medications inhibit metabolizing enzymes, thereby increasing levels of atomoxetine.	• Instruct clients and families to watch for and report increased adverse reactions of atomoxetine. • Concurrent use may require a reduction in the dosage of atomoxetine.

Nursing Administration

- Note any changes in clients related to dosing and timing of medications.

- Administer the medication in one daily dose in the morning or in two divided doses, morning and afternoon, with or without food.

- Instruct clients that therapeutic effect may take 1 to 3 weeks to fully develop.

Nursing Evaluation of Medication Effectiveness

- Depending on therapeutic intent, effectiveness may be evidenced by:

  ○ Improvement of the symptoms of ADHD, such as increase in ability to focus and complete tasks, interact with peers, and manage impulsivity.

MEDICATION CLASSIFICATION: ANTIPSYCHOTICS – ATYPICAL

- Select Prototype Medication: risperidone (Risperdal)
- Other Medications
  - Olanzapine (Zyprexa)
  - Quetiapine (Seroquel)

Purpose

- Expected Pharmacological Action
  - These antipsychotic agents work mainly by blocking serotonin, and to a lesser degree, dopamine receptors. These medications also block receptors for norepinephrine, histamine, and acetylcholine.
- Therapeutic Uses
  - Pervasive development disorders (PDD), including autistic disorder
  - Conduct disorder
  - PTSD
  - Relief of psychotic symptoms

Complications

SIDE/ADVERSE EFFECTS	NURSING INTERVENTIONS/CLIENT EDUCATION
Onset of diabetes mellitus or loss of glucose control in clients with diabetes	• Obtain the client's baseline fasting blood glucose level, and monitor periodically throughout treatment. • Instruct clients and families to report symptoms such as increased thirst, urination, and appetite.
Weight gain	• Advise clients to follow a healthy, low-calorie diet, engage in regular exercise, and monitor weight gain.
Hypercholesterolemia with increased risk for hypertension and other cardiovascular disease	• Monitor cholesterol, triglycerides, and blood glucose if weight gain is more than 14 kg (30.8 lb).
Orthostatic hypotension	• Monitor blood pressure with first dose, and instruct clients to change positions slowly if orthostatic hypotension occurs.
Anticholinergic effects (urinary retention or hesitancy, dry mouth)	• Monitor for these adverse effects, and report their occurrence to the provider. • Encourage clients to use measures to relieve dry mouth (sipping fluids throughout the day).
Symptoms of agitation, dizziness, sedation, and sleep disruption	• Administer an alternative medication if prescribed.
Mild extrapyramidal side effects (EPS), such as tremors	• Monitor for and instruct clients and families to recognize EPS. These effects are usually dose related.

(S) Contraindications/Precautions

- Clients should avoid the use of alcohol.

- Use cautiously in clients with cardiovascular disease, seizures, or diabetes mellitus. Obtain baseline fasting blood glucose levels for clients with diabetes mellitus, and monitor blood glucose level closely.

Interactions

MEDICATION/FOOD INTERACTIONS	NURSING INTERVENTIONS/CLIENT EDUCATION
CNS depressants – Additive CNS depression occurs with concurrent use of alcohol, opioids, or antihistamines.	• Advise clients to avoid alcohol. • Advise clients to avoid hazardous activities (driving).
Barbiturates and phenytoin (Dilantin) promote hepatic drug-metabolizing enzymes, thereby decreasing drug levels of quetiapine.	• Monitor medication for effectiveness.
Fluconazole (Diflucan) inhibits hepatic drug-metabolizing enzymes, thereby increasing drug levels of aripiprazole, quetiapine, and ziprasidone.	• Monitor clients for adverse medication effects.

Nursing Administration

- Administer by oral or IM route (risperidone and olanzapine).

- Advise clients that low doses of medication are given initially and are then gradually increased.

Nursing Evaluation of Medication Effectiveness

- Effectiveness for clients diagnosed with PDD may be evidenced by:

  o Reduction of hyperactivity.

  o Improvement in mood.

- Effectiveness for clients diagnosed with conduct disorder may be evidenced by:

  o Decreased aggressiveness.

- Effectiveness for clients diagnosed with PTSD may be evidenced by:

  ○ Decreased aggressiveness and reduction of flashbacks.

  ○ Improvement of psychotic symptoms (prevention of acute psychotic symptoms, absence of hallucinations, delusions, anxiety, hostility).

  ○ Improvement in ability to perform ADLs.

  ○ Improvement in ability to interact socially with peers.

  ○ Improvement of sleeping and eating habits.

Ⓐ **APPLICATION EXERCISES**

1. A nurse is reinforcing teaching with the parents of a child who has a new prescription for sertraline (Zoloft) about reactions to watch for during the first 3 days of treatment. For which of the following manifestations should the nurse instruct the parents to withhold the medication and notify the provider immediately? (Select all that apply.)

    _____ Diaphoresis

    _____ Incoordination

    _____ Somnolence

    _____ Constipation

    _____ Poor concentration

2. An adolescent has started taking imipramine (Tofranil) to treat depression. Which of the following nursing interventions should the nurse suggest to the adolescent to help minimize an adverse effect of this medication?

    A. Chew sugarless gum.

    B. Wear a mouth guard when sleeping.

    C. Take medication first thing in the morning before eating.

    D. Have between-meal snacks.

3. A nurse is reinforcing teaching with an adolescent who is to start taking buspirone (BuSpar) for an anxiety disorder. Which of the following fluids should the nurse instruct the client to avoid?

    A. Milk

    B. Caffeinated beverages

    C. Grapefruit juice

    D. Carbonated beverages

4. A nurse is caring for a school-age child who has just been prescribed methylphenidate (Daytrana) to treat ADHD. Which of the following should the nurse reinforce with the client and family about the medication?

    A. Apply the patch once daily at bedtime.

    B. Take the oral medication once daily in the morning.

    C. Take the oral medication early in the morning and again at bedtime.

    D. Apply the patch on awakening and remove it at bedtime.

5. A nurse is assisting with the evaluation of an adolescent client who has been taking quetiapine (Seroquel) to help manage PTSD. Which of the following is an indication of the effectiveness of the medication therapy?

    A. Reduction of repetitive behaviors

    B. Clearer memories of the traumatic event

    C. Reduction in attending social events

    D. Improvement in sleeping habits

(A) **APPLICATION EXERCISES ANSWER KEY**

1. A nurse is reinforcing teaching with the parents of a child who has a new prescription for
    sertraline (Zoloft) about reactions to watch for during the first 3 days of treatment. For which of
    the following manifestations should the nurse instruct the parents to withhold the medication
    and notify the provider immediately? (Select all that apply.)

       __X__   **Diaphoresis**

       __X__   **Incoordination**

       _____   Somnolence

       _____   Constipation

       __X__   **Poor concentration**

    **Diaphoresis, incoordination, and poor concentration, as well as fever, hyper-reflexia,
    agitation, and hallucinations are some manifestations of serotonin syndrome, which may
    develop between 2 and 72 hr after beginning treatment with sertraline or other SSRIs.
    The parents should withhold the medication and notify the provider if these symptoms
    develop. Somnolence and constipation are possible effects of SSRIs, but they are not
    indications of serotonin syndrome.**

    (N) NCLEX® Connection: Pharmacological Therapies, Adverse Effects/Contraindications/Side
    Effects/Interactions

2. An adolescent has started taking imipramine (Tofranil) to treat depression. Which of the following
    nursing interventions should the nurse suggest to the adolescent to help minimize an adverse
    effect of this medication?

    A. Chew sugarless gum.

    B. Wear a mouth guard when sleeping.

    C. Take medication first thing in the morning before eating.

    D. Have between-meal snacks.

    **Chewing sugarless gum will help minimize dry mouth, which is an anticholinergic
    effect clients might develop when taking a tricyclic antidepressant medication, such as
    imipramine. Mouth guards are recommended for clients taking medications that are
    known to cause bruxism, such as SSRIs. Taking the medication at bedtime rather than in
    the morning will prevent daytime sleepiness. Following a low-calorie diet plan rather than
    adding extra calories will help prevent weight gain, another common adverse effect.**

    (N) NCLEX® Connection: Pharmacological Therapies, Medication Administration

3. A nurse is reinforcing teaching with an adolescent who is to start taking buspirone (BuSpar) for an anxiety disorder. Which of the following fluids should the nurse instruct the client to avoid?

    A. Milk

    B. Caffeinated beverages

    C. Grapefruit juice

    D. Carbonated beverages

Instruct the client to avoid grapefruit juice because it can increase the effects of buspirone. There are no known interactions between buspirone and milk, caffeinated beverages, or carbonated beverages.

NCLEX® Connection: Pharmacological Therapies, Adverse Effects/Contraindications/Side Effects/Interactions

4. A nurse is caring for a school-age child who has just been prescribed methylphenidate (Daytrana) to treat ADHD. Which of the following should the nurse reinforce with the client and family about the medication?

    A. Apply the patch once daily at bedtime.

    B. Take the oral medication once daily in the morning.

    C. Take the oral medication early in the morning and again at bedtime.

    D. Apply the patch on awakening and remove it at bedtime.

Long-acting methylphenidate (Daytrana) is available as a transdermal patch, which should be applied in the morning and removed after no more than 9 hr each day. Concerta is a long-acting formulation of methylphenidate that should be taken once daily in the morning. Short-acting methylphenidate (Ritalin) is taken orally two or three times daily; however, the last dose is taken no later than late afternoon or early evening to avoid any inference with the child's sleep.

NCLEX® Connection: Pharmacological Therapies, Medication Administration

5. A nurse is assisting with the evaluation of an adolescent client who has been taking quetiapine (Seroquel) to help manage PTSD. Which of the following is an indication of the effectiveness of the medication therapy?

    A. Reduction of repetitive behaviors

    B. Clearer memories of the traumatic event

    C. Reduction in attending social events

    D. Improvement in sleeping habits

Clients who have PTSD typically have difficulty sleeping, and an improvement in sleep patterns is one measure of medication effectiveness. Repetitive behaviors characterize OCD, not PTSD. Clients with PTSD tend to have vivid recollections of the traumatic event and avoid social situations, so these do not indicate an improvement.

NCLEX® Connection: Pharmacological Therapies, Expected Effects

UNIT 4	PSYCHOPHARMACOLOGIC THERAPIES
Chapter 23	Medications for Substance Abuse

Overview

- Abstinence syndrome occurs when a client abruptly withdraws from a drug on which he is physically dependent.

- Symptoms of abstinence syndrome can be distressing and may lead to coma and death.

MAJOR DRUGS OF ABUSE	
SUBSTANCE	**WITHDRAWAL SYMPTOMS**
Alcohol	• Symptoms usually start within 4 to 12 hr of the last intake of alcohol, peak after 24 to 48 hr, and then subside, unless alcohol withdrawal delirium occurs. • Common symptoms include nausea; vomiting; tremors; restlessness and inability to sleep; depressed mood or irritability; increased heart rate, blood pressure, respiratory rate, and temperature; diaphoresis and tonic-clonic seizures may occur, particularly in those prone to seizures. Illusions may also occur. • Alcohol withdrawal delirium may occur 2 to 3 days after cessation of alcohol and last 2 to 3 days. This is considered a medical emergency. Symptoms include severe disorientation, psychotic symptoms (hallucinations), severe hypertension, cardiac dysrhythmias, and delirium. This type of withdrawal may progress to death.
Opioids (heroin, prescription medications)	• Withdrawal symptoms occur within hours to several days after cessation of drug use. • Common symptoms include agitation, insomnia, flu-like symptoms, rhinorrhea, yawning, sweating, and diarrhea. • Withdrawal symptoms are not life threatening, although suicidal ideation may occur.
Nicotine	• Abstinence syndrome is evidenced by irritability, nervousness, restlessness, insomnia, and difficulty concentrating.

MEDICATIONS TO SUPPORT WITHDRAWAL/ABSTINENCE FROM ALCOHOL

Detoxification

INTENDED EFFECTS	NURSING INTERVENTIONS/CLIENT EDUCATION
Benzodiazepines (chlordiazepoxide [Librium], diazepam [Valium], lorazepam [Ativan])	
• Maintenance of the client's vital signs within normal limits • Decrease in the risk of seizures • Decrease in the intensity of withdrawal symptoms	• Administer around the clock or PRN. • Obtain the client's baseline vital signs. • Monitor the client's vital signs and neurological status on an ongoing basis. • Provide for seizure precautions (padded side rails, suction equipment at bedside).
Adjunct Medications (carbamazepine [Tegretol], clonidine [Catapres], propranolol [Inderal])	
• Decrease in seizures – Carbamazepine • Depression of autonomic response (decrease in blood pressure, heart rate, diaphoresis) – Clonidine and propranolol • Decrease in craving – Propranolol	• Provide for seizure precautions (padded side rails, suction equipment at bedside). • Obtain the client's baseline vital signs and continue to monitor on a regular basis.

Abstinence Maintenance (Following Detoxification)

INTENDED EFFECTS	NURSING INTERVENTIONS/CLIENT EDUCATION
Disulfiram (Antabuse)	
• Disulfiram is a daily oral medication that is a type of aversion (behavioral) therapy. • Using disulfiram concurrently with alcohol will cause acetaldehyde syndrome to occur. ○ Effects include nausea, vomiting, weakness, sweating, palpitations, and hypotension. • Acetaldehyde syndrome can progress to respiratory depression, cardiovascular suppression, seizures, and death.	• Inform clients of the potential dangers of drinking any alcohol. • Advise clients to avoid any products that contain alcohol (cough syrups, aftershave lotion). • Encourage clients to wear a medical alert bracelet. • Encourage clients to participate in a 12-step program. • Advise clients that medication effects, such as the potential for acetaldehyde syndrome with alcohol ingestion, persist for 2 weeks following discontinuation of disulfiram.

INTENDED EFFECTS	NURSING INTERVENTIONS/CLIENT EDUCATION
Naltrexone (ReVia)	
• Naltrexone is a pure opioid antagonist that suppresses the craving and pleasurable effects of alcohol (also used for opioid withdrawal).	• Obtain an accurate history to determine if the client is also dependent on opioids. Use of naltrexone will initiate withdrawal syndrome. • Advise clients to take naltrexone with meals to decrease gastrointestinal distress. • Suggest monthly IM injections for clients who have difficulty adhering to the medication regimen.
Acamprosate (Campral)	
Acamprosate decreases unpleasant effects resulting from abstinence (anxiety, restlessness).	• Inform clients that diarrhea may result. • Advise clients to maintain adequate fluid intake and to get adequate rest. • Advise clients to avoid use during pregnancy.

MEDICATIONS TO SUPPORT WITHDRAWAL/ABSTINENCE FROM OPIOIDS

INTENDED EFFECTS	NURSING INTERVENTIONS/CLIENT EDUCATION
Methadone (Dolophine)	
• Methadone is an oral opioid agonist that replaces the opioid to which clients are addicted. This will prevent abstinence syndrome from occurring and remove the need for clients to obtain illegal drugs. • Use for withdrawal and long-term maintenance. Dependence will be transferred from the illegal opioid to methadone.	• Inform clients that the methadone dose must be slowly tapered during detoxification. • Encourage clients to participate in a 12-step program. • Inform clients that they must receive the medication from an approved treatment center.
Clonidine (Catapres)	
• Clonidine assists with withdrawal symptoms related to autonomic hyperactivity (diarrhea, nausea, vomiting). • Clonidine therapy does not reduce the craving for opioids.	• Obtain baseline vital signs. • Advise clients to avoid activities that require mental alertness until symptoms of drowsiness subside. • Encourage clients to chew on gum or hard candy and to sip on small amounts of water or suck on ice chips to treat dry mouth.

INTENDED EFFECTS	NURSING INTERVENTIONS/CLIENT EDUCATION
Buprenorphine (Subutex), Buprenorphine Combined with Naloxone (Suboxone)	
• These medications are agonist-antagonist opioids used for both detoxification and maintenance. • These medications decrease feelings of craving and may be effective in maintaining compliance.	• Inform clients that the medication must be administered from an approved treatment center. • Administer the medications sublingually.

MEDICATIONS TO SUPPORT WITHDRAWAL/ABSTINENCE FROM NICOTINE

INTENDED EFFECTS	NURSING INTERVENTIONS/CLIENT EDUCATION
Bupropion HCL (Wellbutrin, Zyban)	
Bupropion decreases nicotine craving and symptoms of withdrawal.	• To treat dry mouth, encourage clients to chew on gum or hard candy and to sip on small amounts of water or suck on ice chips. • Advise clients to avoid caffeine and other CNS stimulants to control insomnia.
Nicotine Replacement Therapy (nicotine gum [Nicorette], nicotine patch [Nicotrol])	

These nicotine replacements are pharmaceutical product substitutes for the nicotine in cigarettes or chewing tobacco.	• Instruct clients to avoid using any nicotine products while pregnant or breastfeeding.
	• For use of nicotine gum advise clients:
	  ○ That use of chewing gum is not recommended for longer than 6 months.
	  ○ To chew gum slowly and intermittently over 30 min.
	  ○ To avoid eating or drinking 15 min prior to and while chewing the gum.
	• For use of a nicotine patch, advise clients to:
	  ○ Apply a nicotine patch to an area of clean, dry skin each day.
	  ○ Avoid using any nicotine products while wearing the patch.
	  ○ Follow product directions for dosage times.
	  ○ Remove the patch and notify the provider if a local skin reaction occurs.
	  ○ Remove the patch prior to an MRI scan.

Nursing Evaluation of Medication Effectiveness

- Depending on therapeutic intent, effectiveness may be evidenced by:

    ○ Absence of injury.

    ○ Ongoing abstinence from the substance.

    ○ Regular attendance at a 12-step program.

Ⓐ APPLICATION EXERCISES

1. A nurse is caring for a client who is withdrawing from alcohol. Which of the following manifestations should the nurse expect to find when collecting data from the client? (Select all that apply.)

    _____ Nausea

    _____ Somnolence

    _____ Tremors

    _____ Bradycardia

    _____ Diaphoresis

2. Which of the following medications may be used for long-term management of abstinence from alcohol? (Select all that apply.)

    _____ Propranolol (Inderal)

    _____ Chlordiazepoxide (Librium)

    _____ Disulfiram (Antabuse)

    _____ Naltrexone (ReVia)

    _____ Carbamazepine (Tegretol)

3. A nurse is reinforcing teaching to a client who is prescribed clonidine (Catapres) to assist with the maintenance of abstinence from opioids. The nurse should instruct the client to observe for which of the following side effects?

    A. Pallor

    B. Dry mouth

    C. Photosensitivity

    D. Weight loss

4. Match the treatment goal with the appropriate medication.

    _____ Alcohol withdrawal   A. Clonidine (Catapres)

    _____ Heroin withdrawal   B. Naloxone (Narcan)

    _____ Nicotine withdrawal   C. Bupropion (Zyban)

    _____ Alcohol abstinence   D. Lorazepam (Ativan)

    _____ Morphine overdose   E. Naltrexone (Re Via)

APPLICATION EXERCISES ANSWER KEY

1. A nurse is caring for a client who is withdrawing from alcohol. Which of the following manifestations should the nurse expect to find when collecting data from the client? (Select all that apply.)

    <u>__X__</u>   **Nausea**

    _____   Somnolence

    <u>__X__</u>   **Tremors**

    _____   Bradycardia

    <u>__X__</u>   **Diaphoresis**

    Acute alcohol withdrawal is characterized by nausea; vomiting; tremors; restlessness; insomnia (not somnolence); depressed mood or irritability; seizures; elevations in heart rate, respiratory rate, blood pressure, and temperature; and diaphoresis.

    Ⓝ NCLEX® Connection: Psychosocial Integrity, Chemical and other Dependencies

2. Which of the following medications may be used for long-term management of abstinence from alcohol? (Select all that apply.)

    _____   Propranolol (Inderal)

    _____   Chlordiazepoxide (Librium)

    <u>__X__</u>   **Disulfiram (Antabuse)**

    <u>__X__</u>   **Naltrexone (ReVia)**

    _____   Carbamazepine (Tegretol)

    Disulfiram is administered to help the client maintain abstinence from alcohol. If the client drinks alcohol while taking disulfiram, he may experience a mild reaction, such as nausea and vomiting, or a more severe reaction that can lead to respiratory depression and death. Naltrexone is a pure opioid antagonist that suppresses the craving for and pleasurable effects of alcohol. Use propranolol, chlordiazepoxide, and carbamazepine on a short-term basis during detoxification.

    Ⓝ NCLEX® Connection: Pharmacological Therapies, Expected Actions/Outcomes

3. A nurse is reinforcing teaching to a client who is prescribed clonidine (Catapres) to assist with the maintenance of abstinence from opioids. The nurse should instruct the client to observe for which of the following side effects?

    A. Pallor

    B. Dry mouth

    C. Photosensitivity

    D. Weight loss

    Dry mouth is a common side effect of clonidine and the client can manage this by chewing gum or sipping water throughout the day. Clonidine may cause flushing (not pallor), and weight gain (not weight loss) due to sodium retention. Photosensitivity is not associated with clonidine use.

    NCLEX® Connection: Pharmacological Therapies, Adverse Effects/Contraindications/Side Effects/Interactions

4. Match the treatment goal with the appropriate medication.

__D__	Alcohol withdrawal	A. Clonidine (Catapres)
__A__	Heroin withdrawal	B. Naloxone (Narcan)
__C__	Nicotine withdrawal	C. Bupropion (Zyban)
__E__	Alcohol abstinence	D. Lorazepam (Ativan)
__B__	Morphine overdose	E. Naltrexone (Re Via)

    NCLEX® Connection: Pharmacological Therapies, Expected Actions/Outcomes

UNIT 5: SPECIAL POPULATIONS

- Care of Those Who are Dying and/or Grieving

- Mental Health Issues of the Child and Adolescent

NCLEX® CONNECTIONS

When reviewing the chapters in this section, keep in mind the relevant sections of the NCLEX® outline, in particular:

CLIENT NEEDS: PSYCHOSOCIAL INTEGRITY

Relevant topics/tasks include:
- End of Life Care
  - Identify client ability to cope with end of life interventions.
- Grief and Loss
  - Support the client in anticipatory grieving.
- Mental Health Concepts
  - Recognize change in client mental status.
  - Assist in promoting client independence.

UNIT 5   SPECIAL POPULATIONS

Chapter 24   Care of Those Who are Dying and/or Grieving

Ⓐ Overview

- Clients experience loss in many aspects of their lives.

- Grief is the inner emotional response to loss and is exhibited in as many ways as there are individuals.

- Bereavement includes both grief and mourning (the outward display of loss) as an individual deals with the death of a significant individual.

- Palliative, or end-of-life care, is an important aspect of nursing care that attempts to meet the client's physical and psychosocial needs.

- End-of-life issues include decision making in a highly stressful time, during which nurses must consider the desires of clients and families. Any decisions must be shared with other health care personnel for continuity of care during this time of stress, grief, and bereavement.

- Advance directives – Legal documents that direct end-of-life issues

  o   Living wills – Directive documents for medical treatment per a client's wishes

  o   Durable power of attorney for health care – A document that appoints an individual to make medical decisions when a client is no longer able to do so on his own behalf

TYPES OF LOSS	
Necessary loss	Part of the cycle of life; anticipated, but may still be experienced intensely
Actual loss	Any loss of a valued person or item
Perceived loss	Any loss defined by a client that is not obvious to others
Maturational loss	Losses normally expected due to the developmental processes of life
Situational loss	Unanticipated loss caused by an external event

Theories of Grief

- Kübler-Ross: Five Stages of Grief – Stages may not be experienced in order, and the length of each stage will vary from person to person.

  o Denial – Clients have difficulty believing a terminal diagnosis or loss.

  o Anger – Clients lash out at other people or things.

  o Bargaining – Clients negotiate for more time or a cure.

  o Depression – Clients are saddened over the inability to change the situation.

  o Acceptance – Clients accept what is happening and plan for the future.

- Worden: Four Tasks of Mourning – Completion of all four tasks generally takes about a year, but this may also vary from person to person.

  o Task I – Accepting the inevitability of the loss

  o Task II – Using coping mechanisms to experience the emotional pain of the loss

  o Task III – Changing the environment to accommodate the absence of the deceased

  o Task IV – Reallocating emotional ties to new individuals, and moving thoughts about the deceased to a less prominent place in everyday thoughts

Factors Influencing Loss, Grief, and Coping Ability

- An individual's current stage of development

- Interpersonal relationships and social support network

- Type and significance of the loss

- Culture and ethnicity

- Spiritual and religious beliefs and practices

- Prior experience with loss

- Socioeconomic status

- Dysfunctional grieving risks

  o Being dependent upon the deceased

  o Unexpected death at a young age, through violence, or by a socially unacceptable manner

  o Inadequate coping skills or lack of social support

  o Pre-existing mental health issues (depression, substance abuse)

Data Collection

TYPES OF GRIEF	
Normal grief	• This grief is considered uncomplicated. • Emotions may be negative (anger, resentment, withdrawal, hopelessness, guilt), but should change to acceptance of the loss with time. • Some acceptance should be evident by 6 months after the loss, such as being able to talk about the loss and having renewed energy. • Somatic complaints may include chest pain, palpitations, headaches, nausea, changes in sleep patterns, or fatigue.
Anticipatory grief	• This grief implies the "letting go" of an object or person before the loss, as in the case of a terminal illness. • Clients have the opportunity to grieve before the actual loss.
Dysfunctional grief	• This grief involves difficult progression through the expected stages of the grieving process. • Usually the work of grief is prolonged, the clinical findings are more severe, and they may result in depression or exacerbation of a pre-existing disorder. • Clients may have intense feelings of guilt, lowered self-esteem, and suicidal ideation. • Somatic complaints persist for an extended period of time.
Disenfranchised grief	• This grief is an experienced loss that cannot be publicly shared or is not socially acceptable, such as the loss of a loved one through suicide.

Nursing Interventions

- Facilitate Mourning

  - Provide time for the grieving process.

  - Identify expected grieving behaviors (crying, somatic manifestations, anxiety).

  - Use therapeutic communication. Name the emotion that the client is feeling. For example, a nurse may say, "You sound as though you are angry. Anger is a normal feeling for someone who has lost a loved one. Tell me about how you are feeling."

  - Avoid communication that inhibits open expression of feelings, such as offering false reassurance, giving advice, changing the subject, and taking the focus away from the individual who is grieving.

  - Assist clients to accept the reality of the loss.

  - Support the client's efforts to "move on" in the face of the loss.

  - Encourage the building of new relationships as the client is able.

  - Provide continuing support; encourage the support of family and friends.

  - Look for signs of ineffective coping, such as a client refusing to leave her home months after her spouse has died.

- ○ Share information about mourning and grieving with clients who may not realize that feelings such as anger toward the deceased are expected.

- ○ Request a referral for psychotherapy for clients who are having difficulty resolving grief.

- ○ Encourage clients who are grieving to attend a bereavement or grief support group.

- ○ Provide information on available community resources.

- ○ Ask clients if contacting a spiritual adviser would be acceptable, or encourage clients to do so.

- ○ Participate in debriefing provided by professional grief and mental health counselors.

 View Media Supplement: Caring for Those Who are Grieving or Dying (Video)

Client Outcomes

- The client verbalizes needs to the care provider.

- The client begins progressing through the stages of grief in a timely manner.

PALLIATIVE CARE

Overview

- Nurses serve as advocates for a client's sense of dignity and self-esteem by providing palliative care at the end of life.

- Palliative care improves the quality of life of clients and their families facing end-of-life issues.

- Palliative care interventions are used primarily when caring for clients who are dying and family members who are grieving.

- An interdisciplinary team provides palliative care

    - ○ Physicians

    - ○ Nurses

    - ○ Social workers

    - ○ Massage therapists

    - ○ Occupational therapists

    - ○ Music and art therapists

    - ○ Touch and energy therapists

    - ○ Clergy

- Hospice care is a comprehensive care delivery system for the terminally ill that is usually implemented when clients are not expected to live longer than 6 months. Further medical care aimed toward a cure is discontinued, and the focus becomes symptom relief and maintaining the client's quality of life.

Data Collection

CHARACTERISTICS OF DISCOMFORT	SIGNS AND SYMPTOMS OF APPROACHING DEATH
<ul><li>Pain</li><li>Anxiety</li><li>Dyspnea</li><li>Nausea or vomiting</li><li>Dehydration</li><li>Diarrhea or constipation</li><li>Urinary incontinence</li><li>Inability to perform ADLs</li></ul>	<ul><li>Decreased level of consciousness</li><li>Muscle relaxation</li><li>Labored breathing (dyspnea, apnea, Cheyne-Stokes respirations)</li><li>Mucus collection in large airways</li><li>Incontinence of bowel or bladder</li><li>Occurrence of mottling with poor circulation</li><li>Nonreactive pupils</li><li>Weak pulse and dropping blood pressure</li><li>Cool extremities</li><li>Perspiration</li><li>Decreased urine output</li><li>Inability to swallow</li></ul>

- Determine the client's sources of strength and hope.

- Identify the desires and expectations of clients and families for end-of-life care.

Nursing Interventions

- Promote continuity of care and communication by limiting assigned staff changes.

- Assist clients and families to set priorities for end-of-life care.

- Physical Care

    o Give priority to the control of clinical manifestations.

    o Administer medications that manage pain, air hunger, and anxiety.

    o Perform ongoing data collection to determine effectiveness of treatment and need for modifications of treatment plan, such as lower or higher doses of medications.

    o Manage side effects of medications.

    o Reposition clients to maintain airway and comfort.

    o Maintain integrity of skin and mucous membranes.

- Provide an environment that promotes dignity and self-esteem.

  - Remove products of elimination as soon as possible to maintain a clean and odor-free environment.

  - Provide comfortable clothing.

  - Provide grooming for hair, nails, and skin.

  - Encourage family members to bring in possessions that are meaningful to clients, such as pictures.

- Encourage use of relaxation techniques (guided imagery and music).

- Promote decision making in food selection, activities, and health care to involve the client as much control as possible.

- Encourage the client to perform ADLs if the ability and desire exist.

- Psychosocial Care

  - Use trained volunteers when appropriate to provide nonmedical care.

  - Use therapeutic communication to develop and maintain a nurse-client relationship.

  - Facilitate understanding of information regarding disease progression and treatment choices.

  - Facilitate communication between clients, families, and providers.

  - Encourage clients to participate in religious practices that bring comfort and strength, if appropriate.

  - Assist clients in clarifying personal values to facilitate effective decision making.

  - Encourage clients to use coping mechanisms that have worked in the past.

  - Be sensitive to comments made in the presence of clients who are unconscious, as hearing is the last of the senses that is lost.

- Prevention of Abandonment and Isolation

  - Prevent the fear of dying alone.

    - Make presence known by answering call lights in a timely manner and making frequent contact.

    - Enter client's room and speak to the client regularly even if there has not been a request.

    - Keep clients informed of procedure and assessment times.

    - Allow family members to spend the night.

- Support for the Grieving Family

  - Suggest that family members plan visits in a manner that promotes client rest.

  - Ensure that families receive appropriate information as treatment plans change.

- o Provide privacy so family members have the opportunity to communicate and express feelings among themselves without including the client.

- o Determine family members' desire to provide physical care. Provide instruction as necessary.

- o Educate families about physical changes to expect as the client moves closer to death.

Client Outcomes

- The client verbalizes that pain and discomfort are controlled.

- The client rests comfortably and exhibits minimal signs of distress.

- The client and family participate in care as much as client and family desires.

POSTMORTEM CARE

Overview

- A nurse is responsible for following federal and state laws regarding requests for organ or tissue donation, obtaining permission for autopsy, certification and appropriate documentation of the death, and providing safe postmortem (after-death) care.

- The client's family now becomes the nurse's primary focus.

Nursing Interventions

- Care of the Body

  - o Provide care with respect and compassion while attending to the desires of the client and family per their cultural, religious, and social practices.

  - o Recognize that the provider certifies the client's death by pronouncing time and documenting therapies used, and actions taken prior to the death.

  - o Preparing the body for viewing

    - Maintain privacy

    - Shave facial hair (if applicable) if desired by the family

    - Remove all tubes and soiled linens, unless organs are to be donated or it is a coroner's case

    - Remove all personal belongings to be given to the family

    - Cleanse and position the body with a pillow under the head, arms outside the sheet and blanket, dentures in place, and eyes closed

    - Apply fresh linens and a gown

- Brush/comb the client's hair, and replace any hair pieces
- Remove excess equipment and linens from the room
- Dim the lights and minimize noise to provide a calm environment
  - Viewing considerations include:
    - Asking the family if they would like to remain with the body, and honoring any decision. This process should not be rushed.
    - Clarifying where the client's personal belongings should go, either with the body or to a designated person
    - Adhering to the same procedures when the deceased is a newborn, while adding the following:
      - Swaddling the infant's body in a clean blanket
      - Transporting the cradled infant in the nurse's arms or in a special infant carrier
      - Offering mementos of the infant (identification bracelets, footprints, cord clamp, lock of hair, photos)
  - Post viewing
    - Apply identification tags according to the facility's policy.
    - Complete documentation.
    - Remain aware of visitor and staff sensibilities during transport.

- Organ Donation
  - Recognize that request for tissue and organ donation must be made by specially trained personnel.
  - Provide support and reinforce education to family members as decisions are being made. Use a private area for any family discussions concerning donation.
  - Be sensitive to cultural and religious influences.
  - Maintain ventilatory and cardiovascular support for vital organ retrieval.

- Autopsy Considerations
  - The provider typically approaches the family about performing an autopsy.
  - The nurse's role is to answer the family's questions and support the family's choices.
  - Autopsies can be conducted to advance scientific knowledge regarding disease processes, which can lead to the development of new therapies.
  - The law may require an autopsy to be performed if the death is due to a homicide or an accident, or if the death occurs within 24 hr of hospital admission.
  - Most facilities require that equipment used during medical intervention (tubes) remain in place if an autopsy is planned.

- Cultural and Religious Beliefs

    o   Identify cultural and religious beliefs of family members.

    o   Be sensitive to these practices when providing postmortem care.

- Documentation and completion of forms following federal and state laws typically includes:

    o   Person pronouncing the death and at what time.

    o   Consideration of and preparation for organ donation.

    o   Disposition of personal articles.

    o   Names of people notified and any decisions made.

    o   Location of identification tags.

    o   Time the body left the facility and the destination.

Care Nurses Who are Grieving

- Caring long-term for clients can create personal attachments for nurses.

- Coping strategies nurses can use include:

    o   Attending the client's funeral.

    o   Communicating in writing to the client's family.

    o   Attending debriefing sessions with colleagues.

    o   Using stress-management techniques.

    o   Talking with a professional counselor.

Ⓐ APPLICATION EXERCISES

Scenario: An older adult client is accompanied by her adult daughter to the community mental health facility. The client's husband was killed in a motor vehicle crash over a year ago. The client reports that she has been unable to continue any of her normal activities. She does not keep the house clean, has experienced long bouts of crying every day, and does not see her old friends. The daughter asks the nurse if her mother's behavior is to be expected at this time.

1. The nurse should respond by recognizing that the findings demonstrated by the client indicate which of the following types of grief?

   A. Normal

   B. Anticipatory

   C. Dysfunctional

   D. Disenfranchised

2. What clinical findings are present to indicate that the client's grief is becoming prolonged?

3. What further data collection should the nurse make at this time?

4. A nurse is caring for a client who is dying. Identify three nursing interventions that the nurse can use to assist the client in maintaining his dignity and self-esteem during end-of-life care.

5. A toddler was brought to the emergency department by rescue squad after having been found unattended in the swimming pool of an apartment complex. Resuscitation was unsuccessful and the child was pronounced dead. The parents arrive several minutes later, as the mother was notified at her job, and the father was home asleep after having worked the night shift. How should the nurse provide support for the parents?

APPLICATION EXERCISES ANSWER KEY

Scenario: An older adult client is accompanied by her adult daughter to the community mental health facility. The client's husband was killed in a motor vehicle crash over a year ago. The client reports that she has been unable to continue any of her normal activities. She does not keep the house clean, has experienced long bouts of crying every day, and does not see her old friends. The daughter asks the nurse if her mother's behavior is to be expected at this time.

1. The nurse should respond by recognizing that the findings demonstrated by the client indicate which of the following types of grief?

    A. Normal

    B. Anticipatory

    C. Dysfunctional

    D. Disenfranchised

    Clients who are unable to carry out the activities of daily living 6 months after the death may be experiencing dysfunctional grief. Normal grief is uncomplicated, and the client demonstrates some acceptance 6 months after the loss. Anticipatory grief is a type of grief that occurs in anticipation of a future loss. Disenfranchised grief is a type of grief that cannot be publicly recognized.

     NCLEX® Connection: Psychosocial Integrity, Grief and Loss

2. What clinical findings are present to indicate that the client's grief is becoming prolonged?

    The client has bouts of crying every day.

    Behavior changes include being too tired to keep house clean and seldom leaving home.

    The client no longer sees her old friends.

     NCLEX® Connection: Psychosocial Integrity, Grief and Loss

3. What further data collection should the nurse make at this time?

    Check the client for suicidal ideation, depression, and anxiety.

     NCLEX® Connection: Psychosocial Integrity, Grief and Loss

4. A nurse is caring for a client who is dying. Identify three nursing interventions that the nurse can use to assist the client in maintaining his dignity and self-esteem during end-of-life care.

>   **Listen to the client's concerns.**
>
>   **Maintain cleanliness and odor control in the client's physical environment.**
>
>   **Allow the client to participate in ADLs, as desired.**
>
>   **Provide personal grooming assistance, as necessary.**
>
>   **Encourage the client to make decisions regarding food selection, activities, and health care.**

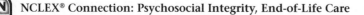 NCLEX® Connection: Psychosocial Integrity, End-of-Life Care

5. A toddler was brought to the emergency department by rescue squad after having been found unattended in the swimming pool of an apartment complex. Resuscitation was unsuccessful and the child was pronounced dead. The parents arrive several minutes later, as the mother was notified at her job, and the father was home asleep after having worked the night shift. How should the nurse provide support for the parents?

>   **Provide time for the parents and family members to be with the child in a private area. The room should be arranged so that it is free of equipment and has adequate seating. The child should be prepared to look as normal as possible. If parents request to hold the child or to take a photograph, assist them to do so. Arrange for the parents to have a lock of their child's hair, clothing, the hospital identification band, or other personal items. Be available to support the parents and answer questions.**

NCLEX® Connection: Psychosocial Integrity, End of Life Concepts

| UNIT 5 | SPECIAL POPULATIONS |
| Chapter 25 | Mental Health Issues of the Child and Adolescent |

Overview

- Mental health and developmental disorders in children and adolescents are not always easily diagnosed, and treatment interventions may be delayed or inadequate. Factors that contribute to this include:

  o Children who do not have the ability or the necessary skills to describe what is happening.

  o Children who demonstrate a wide variation of "normal" behaviors, especially in different developmental stages.

  o Difficulty determining if a child's behavior indicates an emotional problem.

- A child's behavior is problematic when it interferes with home, school, and interactions with peers.

  o Behaviors are considered pathologic when they:

    ▪ Are not age appropriate.

    ▪ Deviate from cultural norms.

    ▪ Create deficits or impairments in adaptive functioning.

- Disorders that may appear during childhood and adolescence

  o Mood disorders (major depressive disorder, dysthymic disorder, bipolar disorder), including suicide

  o Anxiety disorders

  o Substance abuse (the use of cigarettes, alcohol, illegal drugs, prescription medications)

  o Eating disorders, particularly among females

  o Behavioral disorders (ADHD, oppositional defiant disorder, conduct disorder)

  o Pervasive developmental disorders, such as an autistic disorder

- Childhood disorders may have comorbid conditions.

- The characteristics of good mental health for children and adolescents include:

  o Ability to appropriately interpret reality, as well as having a correct perception of the surrounding environment.

  o Positive self-concept.

- o   Ability to cope with stress and anxiety in an age-appropriate way.

- o   Mastery of developmental tasks.

- o   Ability to express oneself spontaneously and creatively.

- o   Ability to develop satisfying relationships.

Data Collection

- General Risk Factors

  - o   Genetic

  - o   Biochemical

  - o   Social and environmental

  - o   Cultural and ethnic

  - o   Degree of resiliency

  - o   Occurrence of trauma or the experiencing of traumatic events in the formative years

MOOD DISORDERS

Overview

- Mood (affective) disorders may occur in childhood. Mood disorders that children are at risk for include major depressive and dysthymic disorders.

Data Collection

- Risk Factors

  - o   Family history of depression

  - o   Physical or sexual abuse or neglect

  - o   Homelessness

  - o   Disputes among parents, conflicts with peers or family, and rejection by peers or family

  - o   Engaging in high-risk behavior

  - o   Learning disabilities

  - o   Having a chronic illness

- Subjective and Objective Data

  - o   Feelings of sadness

  - o   Loss of appetite

  - o   Nonspecific complaints related to health

- o   Engaging in solitary play or work

- o   Changes in appetite resulting in weight changes

- o   Changes in sleeping patterns

- o   Irritability

- o   Aggression

- o   High-risk behavior

- o   Poor school performance or dropping out of school

- o   Difficulty concentrating and/or completing tasks

- o   Feelings of hopelessness about the future

- o   Sense of helplessness

- o   Suicidal tendencies

ANXIETY DISORDERS

Overview

- • An anxiety disorder exists when:

  - o   Anxiety interferes with normal growth and development.

  - o   Anxiety is so serious that the child is unable to function normally at home, in school, and in other areas of life.

- • Separation Anxiety Disorder

  - o   This disorder is characterized by excessive anxiety when a child is separated from or anticipating separation from home or parents. The anxiety may develop into a school phobia or phobia of being left alone. Depression is often a co-occurring disorder.

  - o   Anxiety may progress to a panic disorder or specific phobias.

- • Posttraumatic Stress Disorder (PTSD)

  - o   PTSD may be precipitated by experiencing or seeing a traumatic event.

  - o   Children with PTSD often will respond to the precipitating event in a series of phases. The phases can begin with an arousal that lasts a few minutes to 1 to 2 hr followed by a period of about 2 weeks in which the child will attempt to deal with the event using defense mechanisms. The last phase, lasting for a period of 2 to 3 months, is when the child may develop clinical findings as attempts are made to cope with the event. Failure to cope can lead to obsession regarding the event.

Data Collection

- Risk Factors

    o Anxiety may develop after a specific stressor (death of a relative or pet, illness, move, assault).

- Subjective and Objective Data

    o Children with PTSD may have clinical findings of anxiety, depression, phobia, or conversion reactions.

    o If the anxiety resulting from PTSD is displayed externally, it may be manifested as irritability and aggression with family and friends, poor academic performance, somatic reports, belief that life will be short, and difficulty sleeping.

BEHAVIOR DISORDERS

Overview

- ADHD

    o The inability of a person to control behaviors requiring sustained attention.

    o Types of ADHD

        ▪ Combined type – Most common

        ▪ ADHD predominantly inattentive – Difficulty paying attention, does not appear to listen, easily distracted

        ▪ ADHD predominantly hyperactive-impulsive – Fidgeting, inability to sit still, excessive talking, difficulty waiting for turns, interrupting, disregarding consequences of behavior

    o Inattentive or impulsive behavior may put the child at risk for injury.

    o Behaviors associated with ADHD must be present prior to age 7 and must be present in more than one setting to be diagnosed as ADHD. Behaviors associated with ADHD may receive negative attention from adults and peers.

- Oppositional Defiant Disorder

    o This disorder is characterized by a recurrent pattern of the following antisocial behaviors:

        ▪ Negativity

        ▪ Disobedience

        ▪ Hostility

        ▪ Defiant behaviors (especially toward authority figures)

        ▪ Persistent stubbornness

        ▪ Argumentativeness

- Limit testing
- Unwillingness to compromise
- Refusal to accept responsibility for misbehavior

○ Misbehavior is usually demonstrated at home and directed toward the person best known.

○ Children and adolescents who have oppositional defiant disorder do not see themselves as defiant. They view their behavior as a response to unreasonable demands or circumstances.

○ Children with this behavior disorder may exhibit low self-esteem, mood lability, and a low frustration threshold.

○ Oppositional defiant disorder can develop into conduct disorder.

- Conduct Disorder

CONTRIBUTING FACTORS	MANIFESTATIONS
• Parental rejection and neglect • Difficult infant temperament • Inconsistent child-rearing practices with harsh discipline • Physical or sexual abuse • Lack of supervision • Early institutionalization • Frequent changing of caregivers • Large family size • Association with delinquent peer groups • Parent with a history of psychological illness	• Demonstrates a lack of remorse or care for the feelings of others • Bullies, threatens, and intimidates others • Believes that aggression is justified • Exhibits low self-esteem, irritability, temper outbursts, and reckless behavior • Demonstrates signs of suicidal ideation • Concurrent learning disorders or impairments in cognitive functioning • Demonstrates physical cruelty to others or animals • Has used a weapon that could cause serious injuries • Destroys property of others • Has run away from home • Often lies, shoplifts, and is truant from school

- Pervasive Developmental Disorders

○ Autism spectrum disorder

- A complex neurodevelopmental disorder of unknown etiology with a wide spectrum of behaviors affecting an individual's ability to communicate and interact with others. Cognitive and language development are typically delayed. Characteristic behaviors include inability to maintain eye contact, repetitive actions, and strict observance of routines.

- The disorder is usually observed before 3 years of age.

- There is a wide variability in functioning. Abilities may range from poor (inability to perform self-care, inability to communicate and relate to others) to high (ability to function at near normal levels).

- Other disorders seen in children

  - Mental retardation

    - Below-average intellectual functioning as measured by an IQ of less than 70

  - Learning disorders

    - Group of disorders characterized by difficulty in gaining and using essential skills of listening, speaking, reasoning, performing math, and writing

  - Communication disorders

    - May be expressive, receptive, or a combination of both

    - Treated through a variety of modalities, including speech and language therapies, adaptive communication devices, hearing aids, and sign language

Data Collection

- Subjective and Objective Data

  - In children with behavior disorders, clinical findings generally worsen in:

    - Situations that require sustained attention.

    - Group situations with less structure (playground, classroom activities).

  - Behavioral problems usually occur in school, church, home, and/or recreational activities.

- ADHD

  - Inattention, impulsivity, and hyperactivity are characteristic behaviors of ADHD.

- Autism

  - Physical difficulties experienced by the child with autism may include sensory integration dysfunction, sleep disorders, digestive disorders, feeding disorders, epilepsy, and allergies.

- Mental retardation

  - Significant limitations in communication, self-care, home living, self-direction, social skills, community, work, leisure, academic achievement, health, and safety

Collaborative Care

- Nursing Care

  - Obtain a complete nursing history to include the following:

    - Mother's pregnancy and birth history

    - Sleeping, eating, and elimination patterns; recent weight loss or gain

    - Achievement of developmental milestones

    - Allergies

- Current medications
- Peer and family relationships and school performance
- History of emotional, physical, or sexual abuse
- Parent's perceptions and reactions to the child's behavior
- Family history, including current members of the household
- Substance use/abuse
  - Tobacco products (cigarettes, cigars, snuff, chewing tobacco)
  - Alcohol, frequency of use, driving under the influence, and family history of abuse
  - Drugs (illegal or prescription) used to get high, stay calm, lose weight, or stay awake
- Safety at home and at school
- Actual or potential risk for self-injury
- Presence of depression and suicidal ideation, including a plan, the lethality of that plan, and the means to carry out the plan
- Availability of weapons in the home

○ Perform a complete physical assessment, including a mental status examination.

○ Use primary prevention (education, peer group discussions, mentoring) to decrease risky behavior and to promote healthy behavior and effective coping.

- Work with children to adopt a realistic view of their bodies and to improve overall self-esteem.
- Identify and reinforce the use of positive coping skills.
- Monitor for home safety including proper storage of medications and weapons.
- Emphasize the use of seat belts when in motor vehicles.
- Encourage the use of protective gear for high-impact sports.
- Provide education on contraceptives and other sexual information, such as the transmission and prevention of HIV and other STDs.
- Encourage abstinence, but keep the lines of communication open to allow the adolescent to discuss sexual practices.
- Encourage children and family members to seek professional help, if indicated, and provide resources.

○ Intervene with children who engage in high-risk behaviors.

- Instruct the client and family about factors that contribute to substance dependency and tobacco use. Make appropriate referrals when indicated.
- Inform the client and family about support groups in the community for eating disorders, substance abuse, and general adolescent support.

- Instruct the client regarding individuals within the school environment and community to whom concerns can be voiced about personal safety (police officers, school nurses, counselors, teachers).

- Request referrals to social services when indicated.

- Discuss the use and availability of support hotlines.

  ○ Intervene with children who have anxiety disorders.

- Provide emotional support, accepting use of regression and other defense mechanisms.

- Offer protection during panic levels of anxiety.

- Reinforce cognitive-behavioral therapy techniques such as relaxation and thought stopping.

- Implement methods to increase client self-esteem and feelings of achievement.

- Provide assistance with working through traumatic events or losses to reach an acceptance of what has happened.

- Encourage group therapy.

- Intervene with children who have behavior disorders.

  ○ Use a calm, firm, respectful approach with children.

  ○ Use modeling to demonstrate appropriate behavior.

  ○ Obtain the child's attention before giving directions. Provide short and clear explanations.

  ○ Set clear limits on unacceptable behaviors and be consistent.

  ○ Identify physical activities through which the child can use energy and obtain success.

  ○ Assist parents to develop a reward system using methods such as a wall chart or tokens. Encourage the child to participate.

  ○ Focus on the family and child's strengths, not just the problems.

  ○ Provide a safe environment for the child and others.

  ○ Provide children with specific positive feedback when expectations are met.

  ○ Identify issues that result in power struggles.

  ○ Assist children in developing effective coping mechanisms.

  ○ Encourage children to participate in group, individual, and family therapy.

  ○ Administer medications, such as antipsychotics, mood stabilizers, anticonvulsants, and antidepressants; monitor for side effects.

- Intervene with children who have an autism spectrum disorder.

  ○ Request a referral for early intervention.

  ○ Determine emotional and situational triggers.

- o Provide for a structured environment.

- o Carefully monitor the child's behaviors to ensure safety.

- o Consult with the parents to provide consistent and individualized care.

- o Encourage the parents to participate in planning for and giving care to the child.

- o Use short, concise, concrete, and developmentally appropriate communication.

- o Identify desired behaviors and reward them.

- o Role model social skills.

- o Role play situations that involve conflict.

- o Encourage verbal communication.

- o Limit self-stimulating and ritualistic behaviors by providing alternative play activities.

- o Give plenty of notice before changing routines.

- • Medications

  - o Medications for children and adolescents who have mental health disorders include the selective serotonin reuptake inhibitor, fluoxetine (Prozac); the tricyclic antidepressant, amitriptyline (Elavil); the atypical anxiolytic, buspirone (BuSpar); the atypical antidepressant, bupropion (Wellbutrin); CNS stimulants (methylphenidate [Concerta, Ritalin SR]); and the norepinephrine selective reuptake inhibitor, atomoxetine HCl (Strattera).

- • Interdisciplinary Care

  - o Learning disabilities

    - ▪ An individualized approach depends on the disorder and is generally treated within the school setting as an interdisciplinary method (special education, speech therapy, physical therapy, resource teachers).

  - o Communications disorder

    - ▪ Treated through a variety of modalities (speech and language therapies, adaptive communication devices, hearing aids, sign language)

- • Client Outcomes

  - o The client achieves maximal level of physical, cognitive, and social development.

  - o The client is able to communicate effectively.

  - o The client and family verbalize the need for information and support.

  - o The client verbalizes improved mood.

  - o The client develops realistic goals for the future.

  - o The family identifies strategies for managing disruptive or inappropriate behaviors.

  - o The family identifies strategies for managing long-term care of the client.

Ⓐ APPLICATION EXERCISES

Scenario: A nurse in a provider's office is collecting data from an adolescent who has come to the clinic for her an annual physical. The nurse notices that she makes little eye contact when answering questions and has superficial scratches on her right wrist. The adolescent appears underweight and emotionally distant. She tells the nurse that her parents have recently divorced and that she just moved to a new school district. She also says, "I miss my boyfriend and friends from my old school."

1. Which of the following should the nurse obtain from the adolescent? (Select all that apply.)

    _____ History of weight loss

    _____ Functional ability

    _____ Feelings of safety at home and school

    _____ History of sexual activity

    _____ Substance use (alcohol, drugs, tobacco products)

2. Which of the following findings demonstrated by the adolescent may indicate depression? (Select all that apply.)

    _____ Disobedience

    _____ Inability to concentrate

    _____ Impulsive behavior

    _____ Irritability

    _____ Aggressiveness

3. A school-age child is being evaluated for ADHD. The nurse should expect to find which of the following in this child?

    A. Inability to maintain eye contact

    B. Easily distracted

    C. Anxiety about separation from parent

    D. Self-mutilation

4. A nurse in a provider's office is reinforcing teaching with the parents of a child who has just been diagnosed with ADHD. The nurse should understand that which of the following medications may be prescribed for this child? (Select all that apply.)

    _____ Methylphenidate (Ritalin)

    _____ Thioridazine (Mellaril)

    _____ Molindone (Moban)

    _____ Atomoxetine (Strattera)

    _____ Clozapine (Clozaril)

5. A nurse is observing an adolescent for clinical findings of conduct disorder. The nurse should expect to observe which of the following? (Select all that apply.)

    _____ Hostility

    _____ Frequent lying

    _____ Easy distraction

    _____ Activities that break the law

    _____ Careless mistakes

    _____ Cruelty to neighborhood pets

    _____ Poor eye contact with others

6. A nurse is reinforcing teaching about the clinical findings of autism with the parents of a 4-year-old child. Which of the following findings should the nurse mention in her teaching?

    A. Constant talking to others

    B. Poor language skills

    C. Destructiveness

    D. Reports of somatic problems

Ⓐ APPLICATION EXERCISES ANSWER KEY

Scenario: A nurse in a provider's office is collecting data from an adolescent who has come to the clinic for her an annual physical. The nurse notices that she makes little eye contact when answering questions and has superficial scratches on her right wrist. The adolescent appears underweight and emotionally distant. She tells the nurse that her parents have recently divorced and that she just moved to a new school district. She also says, "I miss my boyfriend and friends from my old school."

1. Which of the following should the nurse obtain from the adolescent? (Select all that apply.)

    __X__ **History of weight loss**

    _____ Functional ability

    __X__ **Feelings of safety at home and school**

    __X__ **History of sexual activity**

    __X__ **Substance use (alcohol, drugs, tobacco products)**

    The nurse should determine the adolescent's risk for a mental health disorder as well as her risk for suicide. Weight loss may be an indication of depression and an eating disorder. The nurse should also inquire about feelings of safety at home and at school, her history of sexual activity, and the use of alcohol, drugs, and tobacco products. All of these factors can influence the mental health of the adolescent. Functional ability should be determined for the older adult client and therefore, is not appropriate for the adolescent.

    Ⓝ NCLEX® Connection: Psychosocial Integrity, Mental Health Concepts

2. Which of the following findings demonstrated by the adolescent may indicate depression? (Select all that apply.)

    _____ Disobedience

    __X__ **Inability to concentrate**

    _____ Impulsive behavior

    __X__ **Irritability**

    __X__ **Aggressiveness**

    Clinical manifestations of depression may include feelings of sadness, inability to concentrate, irritability, and aggressiveness. An adolescent who has oppositional defiant disorder is likely to demonstrate disobedience, and an adolescent who has ADHD is likely to demonstrate impulsive behavior.

    Ⓝ NCLEX® Connection: Psychosocial Integrity, Mental Health Concepts

3. A school-age child is being evaluated for ADHD. The nurse should expect to find which of the following in this child?

   A. Inability to maintain eye contact

   B. Easily distracted

   C. Anxiety about separation from parent

   D. Self-mutilation

   Children with ADHD demonstrate constant movement, are easily distracted, and have difficulty focusing on tasks. Inability to maintain eye contact is a characteristic of a child who has autism. Children who have a separation anxiety disorder become anxious about being separated from their parents. Self-mutilation behavior may occur in a child with posttraumatic stress disorder.

   NCLEX® Connection: Psychosocial Integrity, Mental Health Concepts

4. A nurse in a provider's office is reinforcing teaching with the parents of a child who has just been diagnosed with ADHD. The nurse should understand that which of the following medications may be prescribed for this child? (Select all that apply.)

X	**Methylphenidate (Ritalin)**
	Thioridazine (Mellaril)
	Molindone (Moban)
X	**Atomoxetine (Strattera)**
	Clozapine (Clozaril)

   Children with ADHD may be prescribed methylphenidate, which is a psychostimulant that is used to treat ADHD, or atomoxetine, which is a nonstimulant selective norepinephrine reuptake inhibitor. Thioridazine, molindone, and clozapine are used to treat psychoses.

   NCLEX® Connection: Pharmacological Therapies, Expected Actions/Outcomes

5. A nurse is observing an adolescent for clinical findings of conduct disorder. The nurse should expect to observe which of the following? (Select all that apply.)

X	**Hostility**
X	**Frequent lying**
_____	Easy distraction
X	**Activities that break the law**
_____	Careless mistakes
X	**Cruelty to neighborhood pets**
_____	Poor eye contact with others

Hostility, frequent lying, breaking laws, and cruelty to animals are all manifestations of a conduct disorder. Being easily distracted and making careless mistakes are more likely related to ADHD. Poor eye contact is moreover a manifestation of a pervasive developmental disorder, such as an autistic disorder.

 NCLEX® Connection: Psychosocial Integrity, Mental Health Concepts

6. A nurse is reinforcing teaching about the clinical findings of autism with the parents of a 4-year-old child. Which of the following findings should the nurse mention in her teaching?

A. Constant talking to others

B. Poor language skills

C. Destructiveness

D. Reports of somatic problems

Children with autism have difficulty learning language skills, which may lead to a failure to develop interpersonal relationships. Constant talking to others is a clinical finding of ADHD. Destructiveness is seen in children who have a conduct disorder, and reports of somatic problems is a clinical finding of posttraumatic stress disorder.

 NCLEX® Connection: Psychosocial Integrity, Mental Health Concepts

UNIT 6: PSYCHIATRIC EMERGENCIES

- Crisis Management

- Suicide

- Family and Community Violence

NCLEX® CONNECTIONS

When reviewing the chapters in this section, keep in mind the relevant sections of the NCLEX® outline, in particular:

CLIENT NEEDS: PSYCHOSOCIAL INTEGRITY

Relevant topics/tasks include:
- Abuse/Neglect
  - o Identify signs and symptoms of physical, psychological, or financial abuse in client.
  - o Provide safe environment for abused/neglected client.
- Crisis Intervention
  - o Identify client risk for self injury and/or violence.
  - o Encourage client participation in support groups.
- Coping Mechanisms
  - o Identify significant body or lifestyle changes and other stressors that may affect recovery/health maintenance.

UNIT 6	PSYCHIATRIC EMERGENCIES
Chapter 26	Crisis Management

Overview

- A crisis is an acute, time-limited (usually lasting 4 to 6 weeks) event during which a client experiences an emotional response that cannot be managed with the client's normal coping mechanisms.

- Common characteristics

  - Experience of a sudden event with little or no time to prepare

  - Perception of the event as life threatening or at least life disrupting

  - Loss or decrease in communication with significant others

  - Sense of displacement from the familiar

  - An actual or perceived loss

- Types of crises

  - Situational/external – Often unanticipated loss or change experienced in regular life events

  - Maturational/internal – Achieving new developmental stages, which requires learning additional coping mechanisms

  - Adventitious – The occurrence of natural disasters, crimes, or national disasters

Data Collection

- Risk and Protective Factors

  - Accumulation of unresolved losses

  - Current life stressors

  - Concurrent mental and physical health issues

  - Excessive fatigue or pain

  - Age and developmental stage

  - Support system

  - Prior experience with stress or crisis

- Subjective and Objective Data

  o The nursing history should include the:

    ▪ Presence of suicidal or homicidal ideation requiring hospitalization.

    ▪ Client's perception of the precipitating event.

    ▪ Cultural or religious needs of clients.

    ▪ Support system.

    ▪ Present coping skills.

  o Phases of a crisis

PHASE	MANIFESTATIONS
Phase 1	Escalating anxiety from a threat activates increased defense responses.
Phase 2	Anxiety continues escalating as defense responses fail, functioning becomes disorganized, and clients resort to trial-and-error attempts to resolve anxiety.
Phase 3	Trial-and-error methods of resolution fail, and the client's anxiety escalates to severe or panic levels, leading to flight or withdrawal behaviors.
Phase 4	Clients experience overwhelming anxiety that can lead to anguish and apprehension, feelings of powerlessness and being overwhelmed, dissociative symptoms (depersonalization, detachment from reality), depression, confusion, and violence against others or self.

Collaborative Care

- Nursing Care

  o Initial interventions

    ▪ Identify the current problem and intervene to assist with resolution.

    ▪ Take an active, directive role with clients.

    ▪ Help clients set realistic, attainable goals.

  o Provide for client safety.

    ▪ Recommend hospitalization to protect clients with suicidal or homicidal thoughts.

    ▪ Prioritize interventions to address the client's physical needs first.

  o Use strategies to decrease anxiety.

    ▪ Develop a therapeutic nurse-client relationship.

      □ Remain with clients.

      □ Listen and observe.

      □ Make eye contact.

      □ Ask questions related to the client's feelings.

- ☐ Ask questions related to the event.
- ☐ Demonstrate genuineness and caring.
- ☐ Communicate clearly and, if needed, with clear directives.
- ☐ Avoid false reassurance and other nontherapeutic responses.
- ○ Reinforce teaching about relaxation techniques (meditation).
- ○ Encourage use of coping skills (assertiveness training, parenting skills, occupational training).
- ○ Assist clients with the development of the following type of action plan:
  - ■ Short-term, no longer than 24 to 72 hr
  - ■ Focused on the crisis
  - ■ Realistic and manageable
- Medications
  - ○ Administer antianxiety and/or antidepressant medication as prescribed.
- Client Education
  - ○ Encourage the client to use support agencies and other resources.
  - ○ Request a referral for follow-up care.
- Client Outcomes
  - ○ Client is able to make decisions between two or more options.
  - ○ Client is able to manage anxiety with relaxation techniques.
  - ○ Client returns to precrisis level of functioning.
  - ○ Client has learned new coping skills and uses them.

Ⓐ APPLICATION EXERCISES

Scenario: A nurse on a medical surgical unit is caring for a client who was admitted from the emergency unit 24 hr ago. The client was involved in a motor vehicle crash. The client has multiple lacerations, and fractured pelvis and radius. The client's adolescent son was killed in the crash.

1. Which of the following nursing actions has the highest priority?

    A. Evaluate outside support.

    B. Evaluate client safety.

    C. Manage pain.

    D. Provide active listening.

2. What type of crisis did the client experience?

3. Which of the following medications should the nurse anticipate administering to the client?

    A. Lithium carbonate (Lithobid)

    B. Paroxetine (Paxil)

    C. Risperidone (Risperdal)

    D. Haloperidol (Haldol)

4. A nurse is providing emotional support to a client. The client's attempt to resolve the crisis by trial-and-error methods have failed. This manifestation represents which of the following phases of a crisis?

    A. Phase 1

    B. Phase 2

    C. Phase 3

    D. Phase 4

(A) APPLICATION EXERCISES ANSWER KEY

Scenario: A nurse on a medical surgical unit is caring for a client who was admitted from the emergency unit 24 hr ago. The client was involved in a motor vehicle crash. The client has multiple lacerations, and fractured pelvis and radius. The client's adolescent son was killed in the crash.

1. Which of the following nursing actions has the highest priority?

    A. Evaluate outside support.

    B. Evaluate client safety.

    C. Manage pain.

    D. Provide active listening.

    The first priority for a client in crisis is safety. The nurse should evaluate client safety by determining risk for injury, such as suicide. The other nursing actions are important, but not the highest priority at this time.

 NCLEX® Connection: Psychosocial Integrity, Crisis Intervention

2. What type of crisis did the client experience?

    The client experienced a situational crisis. A situational crisis occurs when there is a loss or change experienced in an everyday event, and is often unanticipated. A maturational crisis occurs when the client achieves a new developmental stage that requires new coping mechanisms. An adventitious crisis occurs when there is a disaster such as a hurricane.

 NCLEX® Connection: Psychosocial Integrity, Crisis Intervention

3. Which of the following medications should the nurse anticipate administering to the client?

    A. Lithium carbonate (Lithobid)

    B. Paroxetine (Paxil)

    C. Risperidone (Risperdal)

    D. Haloperidol (Haldol)

    This client may experience depression related to his loss and may receive a prescription for paroxetine, an antidepressant. Mood stabilizers such as lithium are used for bipolar disorder. Antipsychotic medications, such as risperidone and haloperidol, may be prescribed for disturbed thought processes, but usually when accompanied by other psychotic symptoms (hallucinations, delusions, blunt affect). Antipsychotics are not indicated in a short-term crisis situation.

 NCLEX® Connection: Pharmacological Therapies, Expected Effects/Outcomes

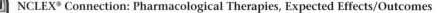

4. A nurse is providing emotional support to a client. The client's attempt to resolve the crisis by trial-and-error methods have failed. This manifestation represents which of the following phases of a crisis?

    A. Phase 1

    B. Phase 2

    C. Phase 3

    D. Phase 4

In Phase 3 of a crisis, trial-and-error methods fail and the client's anxiety level may escalate to panic. In Phase 1, escalating anxiety activates defense responses. In Phase 2, the client attempts to resolve the crisis by trial-and-error methods. In Phase 4, the client is overwhelmed by anxiety, which may lead to depression, confusion, and possible violence against self and others.

(N) **NCLEX® Connection: Psychosocial Integrity, Crisis Intervention**

UNIT 6	PSYCHIATRIC EMERGENCIES
Chapter 27	Suicide

Overview

- Suicide is the intentional act of killing oneself.

- Clients who are suicidal may be ambivalent about death. Intervention can make a difference.

- Clients contemplating suicide believe that the act is the end to problems. Little concern is given to the finality of the act and the ramifications to those left behind. Long-term therapy is needed for the survivors.

- Suicidal ideation occurs when clients are having thoughts about committing suicide.

- Myths regarding suicide include:

  o People who talk about suicide never commit it.

  o People who are suicidal only want to hurt themselves, not others.

  o There is no way to help someone who really wants to kill himself.

  o Mention of the word suicide will cause the suicidal individual to actually commit suicide.

  o Ignoring verbal threats of suicide or challenging a person to carry out suicide plans, will reduce the individual's use of these behaviors.

  o People who talk about suicide are only trying to get attention.

- Levels of Nursing Intervention

  o Primary – Prevention strategies include providing information and education to at-risk populations

  o Secondary – Management of the suicide crisis

Data Collection

- Risk Factors

  o Those at highest risk for suicide include adolescent, young adult, and older adult males; Native Americans as a group; and persons with comorbid mental illness (depressive disorders, anxiety disorders, substance abuse, schizophrenia, personality disorders).

- o Untreated depression increases the risk of suicide in older adult clients. Other risk factors for older adult clients include loss of employment and finances, feelings of isolation, loneliness, powerlessness, prior attempts at suicide (older adult clients are more likely to succeed), change in functional ability, alcohol or other substance abuse, and loss of loved ones.

- o Physiological factors

  - ■ Family history of suicide

  - ■ Physical disorders, such as AIDS, cancer, cardiovascular disease, stroke, chronic renal failure, cirrhosis, dementia, epilepsy, head injury, Huntington's disease, and multiple sclerosis

- o Psychosocial factors

  - ■ Sense of hopelessness

  - ■ Intense emotions, such as rage, anger, or guilt

  - ■ Poor interpersonal relationships at home and work

  - ■ Developmental stressors, such as those experienced by adolescents

- • Protective Factors

  - o Feelings of responsibility toward family

  - o Current pregnancy

  - o Religious and cultural beliefs

  - o Overall satisfaction with life

  - o Presence of adequate social support

  - o Effective coping and problem-solving skills

  - o Intact reality testing

  - o Access to appropriate medical care

- • Subjective Data

  - o Observe carefully for verbal and nonverbal clues. It is important to ask clients if they are thinking of suicide. This will not give clients the idea to commit suicide.

  - o Comments are usually made to someone clients perceive as supportive.

  - o Comments or signals may be overt or covert.

    - ■ Overt comment – "There is just no reason for me to go on living."

    - ■ Covert comment – "Everything is looking pretty grim for me."

- Objective Data

  o Lacerations, scratches, and scars could indicate previous attempts at self-harm.

  o Evaluate the client's suicide plan.

    - How lethal is the plan?

    - Can the client describe the plan exactly?

    - Does the client have access to the intended method?

    - Has the client's mood changed? A sudden change in mood from sad and depressed to happy and peaceful may indicate a client's intention to commit suicide.

    - Has the client's energy level changed? A sudden increase in energy level may be the result of the initial therapeutic effect of the start of an antidepressant medication.

- Standardized Assessment Tool

  o The SAD PERSONS scale is a valuable tool that evaluates 10 major risk factors for suicide and assigns scores for each.

Collaborative Care

- Nursing Care

  o Self-assessment

    - Nurses need to determine how they personally feel about suicide.

    - Nurses need to be comfortable asking questions about suicidal ideation and following up on a client's answers.

    - Death of a client by suicide can cause nurses to experience hopelessness, helplessness, ambivalence, anger, anxiety, avoidance, and denial. Nurses should be encouraged to participate in debriefing sessions with coworkers.

  o Suicide precautions include milieu therapy within the facility.

    - Initiate one-on-one constant supervision around the clock, always having clients in sight, and being physically close.

    - Document the client's location, mood, quoted statements, and behavior every 15 min, or per facility protocol.

    - Remove all glass, metal silverware, electrical cords, vases, belts, shoelaces, metal nail files, tweezers, matches, razors, perfume, shampoo, and plastic bags from the client's room and vicinity.

    - Allow clients to use only plastic eating utensils.

    - Check the environment for possible hazards (windows that open, shower heads, overhead pipes that are easily accessible).

    - During observation periods, always check the client's hands, especially if they are hidden from sight.

- Ensure that clients swallow all medications.

- Identify if the client's current medications can be lethal with overdose. If so, collaborate with the provider to have less dangerous medications substituted, if possible.

- Ensure that visitors are aware of suicide precautions and rules restricting bringing possibly harmful items to the client.

○ Therapeutic communication

- When questioning clients about suicide, always use a follow-up question if the first answer is negative. For example: The client says, "I'm feeling completely hopeless." The nurse says, "Are you thinking of suicide?" Client: "No, I'm just sad." Nurse: "I can see you're very sad. Are you thinking about hurting yourself?" Client: "Well, I've thought about it a lot."

- Establish a trusting therapeutic relationship.

- Limit the amount of time an at-risk client spends alone.

- Involve significant others in the treatment plan.

- Carry out treatment plans for clients with co-occuring disorders (dual diagnosis of substance abuse).

○ Ask clients to agree to a no-suicide contract, which is a verbal or written agreement that clients make to not harm themselves, but instead to seek help.

- Recognize that a no-suicide contract is not legally binding and only use according to agency policy.

- Use a no-suicide contract to develop and maintain trust between the nurse and the client.

- Do not use a no-suicide contract to replace other suicide prevention strategies.

- Do not use no-suicide contracts for clients who are in crisis, under the influence of substances, psychotic, very impulsive, and/or very angry/agitated.

- Medications to prevent suicide

MEDICATION EXAMPLE	NURSING INTERVENTION/CLIENT EDUCATION
Antidepressants: Selective Serotonin Reuptake Inhibitors (SSRIs)	

• Citalopram (Celexa)
• Fluoxetine (Prozac)
• Sertraline (Zoloft)
	• Instruct clients to:
	  ○ Not stop taking the medication suddenly.
	  ○ Avoid hazardous activities (driving, operating heavy equipment/machinery) until medication side effects are known. Side effects may include nausea, headache, and CNS stimulation (agitation, insomnia, anxiety).
	  ○ Follow a healthy diet, as weight gain can occur with long-term use.
	• Monitor for clinical findings of increased depression and intent of suicide.
	• Tell clients that the medication may take 1 to 3 weeks for for initial therapeutic effects and up 2 months for maximal response.
	• Tell clients that sexual dysfunction may occur. Notify the provider if effects are intolerable.

MEDICATION EXAMPLE	NURSING INTERVENTION/CLIENT EDUCATION
Sedative Hypnotic Anxiolytics (Benzodiazepines)	
• Diazepam (Valium) • Lorazepam (Ativan)	• Observe for CNS depression (sedation, lightheadedness, ataxia, decreased cognitive function). • Instruct clients to avoid the use of other CNS depressants (alcohol) and to avoid hazardous activities (driving, operating heavy equipment/machinery). • Tell clients that caffeine interferes with the desired effects of the medication. • Advise clients who have been taking these medications regularly and in high doses not to stop taking them abruptly. The provider will taper the dose over several weeks to prevent withdrawal symptoms.
Mood Stabilizers	

• Lithium carbonate (Eskalith)	• Tell clients that gastrointestinal effects may be minimized by taking medication with food or milk.
	• Recommend that clients:
	  o Maintain a healthy diet and exercise regularly to minimize weight gain.
	  o Maintain fluid intake of 2 to 3 L/day from food and beverage sources.
	  o Maintain adequate sodium intake.
	• Encourage clients to comply with laboratory appointments needed to monitor lithium effectiveness and adverse effects.

Antiepileptics	
• Valproic acid (Depakote)	• Tell clients to take the medication with food to minimize gastrointestinal discomfort.
Atypical Antipsychotics	
• Risperidone (Risperdal) • Olanzapine (Zyprexa)	• Advise clients to maintain a healthy diet and exercise regularly to minimize weight gain. • Instruct clients to report clinical manifestations of agitation, dizziness, sedation, and sleep disruption to the provider, as the medication may need to be changed.

- Care After Discharge
  - Client Education
    - Create a support-system list – Specific names, agencies, and telephone numbers that clients can call for support and in case of an emergency.
    - Encourage clients to adhere to the medication regimen and participate in follow-up care.
- Client Outcomes
  - The client identifies at least two people who can provide emotional support.
  - The client verbalizes a decrease in anxiety.
  - The client remains free from harm.

(A) APPLICATION EXERCISES

Scenario: A nurse is caring for an adolescent who was admitted involuntarily to an acute care mental health facility.

1. Which of the following factors places the adolescent at risk for suicide? (Select all that apply.)

    _____ History of bipolar disorder

    _____ Family history of suicide

    _____ History of substance abuse

    _____ Religious background

    _____ Young adult

2. The nurse and the adolescent are standing near a window on the sixth floor of the mental health facility. The adolescent is lucid with no sign of psychosis today and remarks, "I wonder if anyone has ever jumped from up here." The nurse asks the adolescent if he is thinking about suicide and he replies "No." Which of the following actions should the nurse take next?

    A. Rephrase the question and ask the adolescent again.

    B. Place the adolescent in one-to-one observation.

    C. Ask the adolescent to sign a no-suicide contract.

    D. Encourage the adolescent to identify the major stressors in his life.

3. A client who has depression shows willingness to talk to the nurse about current feelings but states, "I'll talk to you, but please don't tell anyone else what I am going to tell you! Will you promise me?" Which of the following responses by the nurse is appropriate?

    A. "What did you talk about in therapy this week?"

    B. "I am so pleased that you are working on your problems."

    C. "I cannot keep a secret that is related to your safety and well-being."

    D. "Would you rather talk to your mental health counselor about your problem?"

4. A nurse is assisting with the orientation of a new employee. The SAD PERSONS tool is being used to evaluate a client's current status. The nurse explains to the employee that the purpose of this tool is to determine the client's

    A. Ability to cope

    B. Problem-solving ability

    C. Suicide potential

    D. Anxiety level

5. A nurse is caring for a client who says, "I plan to commit suicide." Which of the following findings is the nurse's priority?

   A. Client's educational and economic background

   B. Lethality of method and availability of means

   C. Quality of the client's social support

   D. Client's insight into the reasons for the decision

(A) **APPLICATION EXERCISES ANSWER KEY**

Scenario: A nurse is caring for an adolescent who was admitted involuntarily to an acute care mental health facility.

1. Which of the following factors places the adolescent at risk for suicide? (Select all that apply.)

   __X__ **History of bipolar disorder**

   __X__ **Family history of suicide**

   __X__ **History of substance abuse**

   _____ Religious background

   __X__ **Young adult**

   A history of a mood disorder such as bipolar disorder, a family history of suicide, and a history of substance abuse places the adolescent at greater risk for suicide. Adolescents and young adults are at the greatest risk for suicide. A strong religious background may reduce the client's risk for suicide.

(N) NCLEX® Connection: Psychosocial Integrity, Crisis Intervention

2. The nurse and the adolescent are standing near a window on the sixth floor of the mental health facility. The adolescent is lucid with no sign of psychosis today and remarks, "I wonder if anyone has ever jumped from up here." The nurse asks the adolescent if he is thinking about suicide and he replies "No." Which of the following actions should the nurse take next?

   A. Rephrase the question and ask the adolescent again.

   B. Place the adolescent in one-to-one observation.

   C. Ask the adolescent to sign a no-suicide contract.

   D. Encourage the adolescent to identify the major stressors in his life.

   Using the nursing process, the next action the nurse should take is to collect more data by asking the adolescent the question again. Placing him in one-to-one observation, asking him to sign a no-suicide contract, and encouraging him to identify the major stressors in his life are important; however, this is not the next action the nurse should take.

(N) NCLEX® Connection: Psychosocial Integrity, Crisis Intervention

3. A client who has depression shows willingness to talk to the nurse about current feelings but states, "I'll talk to you, but please don't tell anyone else what I am going to tell you! Will you promise me?" Which of the following responses by the nurse is appropriate?

    A. "What did you talk about in therapy this week?"

    B. "I am so pleased that you are working on your problems."

    C. "I cannot keep a secret that is related to your safety and well-being."

    D. "Would you rather talk to your mental health counselor about your problem?"

    The nurse should tell the client that she cannot keep a secret that is related to the client's safety and well-being. The nurse is required to talk to the health care team about important issues. Asking the client what he talked about in therapy is nontherapeutic because the nurse has changed the subject. By telling the client that she is pleased, the nurse is giving approval, which is nontherapeutic. Asking the client if he would like to talk to someone else is a way of avoiding the subject and is not conducive to a therapeutic nurse-client relationship.

 NCLEX® Connection: Psychosocial Integrity, Therapeutic Communication

4. A nurse is assisting with the orientation of a new employee. The SAD PERSONS tool is being used to evaluate a client's current status. The nurse explains to the employee that the purpose of this tool is to determine the client's

    A. Ability to cope

    B. Problem-solving ability

    C. Suicide potential

    D. Anxiety level

    The SAD PERSONS tool is used specifically to evaluate the client's potential for committing suicide. Information on the other options are not provided by this tool.

 NCLEX® Connection: Psychosocial Integrity, Crisis Intervention

5. A nurse is caring for a client who says, "I plan to commit suicide." Which of the following findings is the nurse's priority?

    A. Client's educational and economic background

    B. Lethality of method and availability of means

    C. Quality of the client's social support

    D. Client's insight into the reasons for the decision

    The greatest risk to the client is self-harm as a result of carrying out a suicide plan. The nurse's priority is to determine how lethal the method is, how available the method is, and how detailed the plan is. Determining the client's education and economic background, the quality of the client's social support, and the client's insight into the reasons for the decision are all important in caring for the client, but are not the priority at this time.

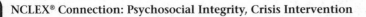 NCLEX® Connection: Psychosocial Integrity, Crisis Intervention

UNIT 6	PSYCHIATRIC EMERGENCIES
Chapter 28	Family and Community Violence

Overview

- Anger, a normal feeling, is an emotional response to frustration as perceived by the individual. It can be positive if there is truly an unfair or wrong situation that needs to be righted.

- Anger becomes negative when it is denied, suppressed, or expressed inappropriately, such as by using aggressive behavior.

  o Denied or suppressed anger can manifest as physical or psychological findings, such as headaches, coronary artery disease, hypertension, gastric ulcers, depression, or low self-esteem.

- Violence by one person toward another is a social act involving a serious abuse of power. Usually, a relatively stronger person controls or injures another, typically the least powerful person accessible to the abuser. This includes acts of violence committed by spouse against spouse, parent against child, child against parent, or stranger against victim.

ANGER MANAGEMENT

Overview

- Aggression

  o Inappropriately expressed anger can become hostility or aggression.

  o Aggression includes physical or verbal responses that indicate rage and potential harm to self, others, or property.

  o Clients who are often angry and aggressive may have underlying feelings of inadequacy, insecurity, guilt, fear, and rejection.

- Comorbidities include depressive disorders, PTSD, Alzheimer's disease, and personality and psychotic disorders.

- Categories of anger and aggressive behavior on a mental health unit

  o Preassaultive – The client becomes angry and exhibits increasing anxiety, hyperactivity, and verbal abuse.

  o Assaultive – The client commits an act of violence. Seclusion and physical restraints may be required.

  o Postassaultive – Staff reviews the incident with the client.

- Despite the potential for anger and aggression among individuals with mental illness, it is important to understand that individuals who are mentally ill are more likely to hurt themselves than to express aggression against others.

Data Collection

- Risk Factors

  o Past history of aggression, poor impulse control, and violence

  o Poor coping skills and limited support systems

  o Comorbidity that leads to acts of violence (psychotic delusions, command hallucinations, cognitive disorders, traumatic brain injury or other CNS disorders)

  o Living in a violent environment

  o Limit setting by the nurse within the therapeutic milieu

- Subjective and Objective Data

  o Hyperactivity, such as pacing or restlessness

  o Defensive response to any criticism

  o Easily offended

  o Eye contact that is intense or lack of eye contact

  o Facial expressions, such as frowning or grimacing

  o Body language, such as clenching fists or waving arms

  o Rapid breathing

  o Aggressive postures, such as leaning forward, appearing tense, or hands on hips

  o Verbal clues, such as loud, rapid talking

  o Drug or alcohol intoxication

Collaborative Care

- Nursing Care

  o Provide a safe environment not only for clients who are aggressive, but also for other clients and staff on the unit.

  o Follow policies of the mental health setting when working with clients who demonstrate aggression.

  o Identify triggers or preconditions that escalate client's emotions.

  o Interventions to handle aggressive and/or escalating behavior in a mental health setting:

    - Respond quickly.

    - Remain calm and in control.

- Encourage clients to express feelings verbally.

- Use therapeutic communication techniques (reflective techniques, silence, active listening).

- Allow clients as much personal space as possible.

- Maintain eye contact and sitting or standing at the same eye level as client.

- Communicate with honesty and sincerity.

- Maintain a nonaggressive stance.

- Avoid accusatory or threatening statements.

- Describe options clearly and offer clients choices.

- Reassure clients that staff are present to help prevent loss of control.

- Set limits for the client:

  □ Tell the client calmly and directly what he must do in a particular situation, such as "I need you to stop yelling and walk with me to the day room where we can talk."

  □ Use physical activity, such as walking, to de-escalate anger and behaviors.

  □ Inform the client of the consequences of his behavior, such as loss of privileges.

- Use pharmacological interventions if clients do not respond to calm limit setting.

- Plan for four to six staff members to be available and in sight of the client as a "show of force" if appropriate.

○ Use seclusion and restraint according to legal guidelines and only as a last resort after other less restrictive options have been tried.

- Seclusion and restraint do not usually lead to positive behavior change. Seclusion and restraint may keep individuals safe during a violent outburst. But the use of restraint itself can be dangerous and has, on rare occasions, led to the death of clients due to reasons such as suffocation and strangulation.

- Remove clients from seclusion or restraint as soon as the crisis is over and when the client attempts reconciliation and is no longer aggressive.

○ Following an aggressive or violent episode:

- Discuss ways for clients to keep control during the aggression cycle.

- Encourage clients to talk about the incident and what triggered and escalated the aggression from the client's perspective.

- Debrief the staff to evaluate the effectiveness of actions.

- Document the entire incident completely by including:

  □ Behaviors leading up to, as well as those observed throughout, the critical incident.

  □ Nursing interventions implemented and the client's response.

- Medications

  o Haloperidol (Haldol)

    ▪ Use haloperidol, an antipsychotic agent, to control aggressive and impulsive behavior.

    ▪ Nursing considerations

      ▫ Monitor for clinical manifestations of Parkinsonian and anticholinergic side effects.

  o Use other medications to prevent violent behavior by treating the underlying disorder. These include antidepressants (SSRIs), mood stabilizers (lithium), and sedative/hypnotic medications (benzodiazepines).

- Care After Discharge

  o Nursing actions

    ▪ Reinforce to clients how to manage medications.

    ▪ Assist clients to develop problem-solving skills.

  o Client education

    ▪ Encourage clients to return for follow-up.

    ▪ Encourage clients to attend a support group.

- Client Outcomes

  o The client recognizes when feelings of anger occur and seeks appropriate assistance from staff.

  o The client takes responsibility for own actions.

  o The client is able to diffuse anger without losing control of behavior.

  o The client demonstrates appropriate problem-solving skills rather than violent behavior.

VIOLENCE

Overview

- Nurses must be prepared to deal with various types of violence and the mental health consequences.

  o Violence may be caused by a family member, a stranger, or an acquaintance. Or it can come from a human-caused, mass-casualty incident, such as a terrorist attack.

  o Natural disasters, such as hurricanes and earthquakes, can cause mental health effects comparable to those attributed to human-caused violence.

  o Violence against a person with mental illness is more likely to occur when factors such as poverty, transient lifestyle, and substance abuse are present.

- A person with mental illness is no more likely to harm strangers than anyone else.
- The factor most likely to cause violence between strangers is a past history of violence and criminal activity.

Data Collection

- Risk Factors
  - The female partner is the victim in the majority of family violence, but the male partner may also be a victim of violence.
  - Victims are at the greatest risk for violence when they try to leave the relationship.
  - Pregnancy tends to increase the likelihood of violence toward the domestic partner. The reason for this is unclear, but could be jealousy or feelings of rejection.
  - Victims of rape include individuals of all ages and can be either male or female.
  - Factors that make abuse against children more likely include:
    - The child is under 3 years of age.
    - The child is perceived by the perpetrator as being different (the child is the result of an unwanted pregnancy, is physically disabled, or has some other trait that makes him particularly vulnerable).
  - Older adults within the home may be abused because they are in poor health, exhibit disruptive behavior, or are dependent on a caregiver. The potential for violence against an older adult is highest in families where violence has already occurred.
  - Violence is most common within family groups, and most violence is aimed at family and friends rather than strangers.
    - Family violence occurs across all economic and educational backgrounds and racial and ethnic groups in the United States and is often termed "maltreatment."
    - Maltreatment can occur against children, domestic partners, or older adult family members.
    - Within the family, a cycle of violence can occur between domestic (intimate) partners:
      - Tension-building phase – The abuser has minor episodes of anger and may be verbally abusive and responsible for some minor physical violence. The victim is tense during this stage and tends to accept the blame for what is happening.
      - Serious battering phase – The tension increases and a serious incident takes place. The victim may try to cover up the injury or may get help.
      - Honeymoon phase – The situation is defused for awhile after the violent episode. The abuser becomes loving, promises to change, and is sorry for the behavior. The victim wants to believe this and hopes for a change. Eventually, the cycle begins again.
      - Periods of escalation and de-escalation usually continue with shorter and shorter periods of time between the two. Repeated episodes of violence lead to feelings of powerlessness.

- ○ Cultural differences can influence how the client responds to interventions, and the appropriateness of nursing interactions with the client.

- Subjective and Objective Data

  - ○ Types of violence

    - ■ Physical violence resulting in pain or harm:

      - □ Toward an infant or child, as is the case with shaken baby syndrome (caused by violent shaking of young infants).

      - □ Toward a domestic partner, such as striking or strangling the partner.

      - □ Toward an older adult in the home (elder abuse), such as pushing an older adult parent and causing her to fall.

    - ■ Sexual violence occurs when sexual contact takes place without consent, whether the victim is able or unable to give consent.

      - □ Rape-trauma syndrome

        - ▸ Acute phase – Occurs immediately following the rape, lasts for about 2 weeks, and consists of the following:

          - ▹ Initial emotional reaction

            - ◆ An expressed reaction is overt and consists of emotional outbursts, including crying, laughing, hysteria, anger, and incoherence.

            - ◆ A controlled reaction is ambiguous. The survivor may appear calm and have blunted affect, but may also be confused, have difficulty making decisions, and feel numb.

          - ▹ A somatic reaction occurs later and lasts about 2 weeks. The client may have a variety of findings, including:

            - ◆ Bruising and soreness from the attack

            - ◆ Muscle tension, headaches, and sleep disturbances

            - ◆ Gastrointestinal findings (nausea, anorexia, diarrhea, abdominal pain)

            - ◆ Genitourinary findings (vaginal pain or discomfort)

            - ◆ A variety of emotional reactions, including embarrassment, a desire for revenge, guilt, anger, fear, anxiety, and denial, all of which are normal reactions

        - ▸ Long-term reorganization phase – Occurs 2 weeks or more after the attack. Long-term psychological effects of sexual assault include:

          - ▹ Flashbacks and other intrusive thoughts about the assault

          - ▹ Increased activity, such as visiting friends frequently or moving residence, due to a fear that the assault will recur

- ▷ Increased emotional responses (crying, anxiety, rapid mood swings)

- ▷ Fears and phobias (fear of being alone, fear of sexual encounters)

- ▷ Difficulties with daily functioning, relationships, low self-esteem, substance abuse, depression, sexual dysfunction, and somatic reports, such as headache or fatigue

- ■ Emotional violence, which includes behavior that minimizes an individual's feelings of self-worth or humiliates, threatens, or intimidates a family member. It often occurs over a very long period of time.

- ■ Neglect, which includes the failure to provide:

  - □ Physical care, such as feeding

  - □ Emotional care, such as interacting with a child, and/or stimulation necessary for a child to develop normally

  - □ An education for a child, such as enrolling a young child in school

  - □ Needed health or dental care, or preventive health and dental care.

- ■ Economic maltreatment, which includes:

  - □ Failure to provide for the needs of a victim when adequate funds are available

  - □ Unpaid bills, resulting in disconnection of heat or electricity

○ Victim characteristics

- ■ Demonstration of low self-esteem and feelings of helplessness, hopelessness, powerlessness, guilt, and shame

- ■ Attempts to protect the perpetrator and accept responsibility for the abuse

- ■ Possible denial of the severity of the situation and feelings of anger and terror

○ Perpetrator characteristics

- ■ Possible use of threats and intimidation to control the victim

- ■ Is usually an extreme disciplinarian who believes in physical punishment

- ■ Possible history of substance abuse

- ■ Is likely to have experienced family violence as a child

○ Infants

- ■ Shaken baby syndrome – Shaking may cause intracranial hemorrhage. Check for respiratory distress, bulging fontanelles, and increased head circumference. Retinal hemorrhage may be present.

- ■ Any bruising on an infant before 6 months of age is suspicious.

- ○ Preschoolers to adolescents
  - Look for unusual bruising, such as on abdomen, back, or buttocks. Bruising is common on arms and legs in these age groups.
  - Look for the mechanism of injury, which may not be congruent with the physical appearance of the injury. Numerous bruises at different stages of healing may indicate continued beatings. Be suspicious of bruises or welts that have taken on the shape of a belt buckle or other object.
  - Look for burns. Burns covering "glove" or "stocking" areas of the hands or feet, and the absence of "splash marks," may indicate forced immersion into boiling water. Small, round burns may be caused by lit cigarettes.
  - Look for fractures with unusual features, such as forearm spiral fractures, which could be caused by twisting the extremity forcefully. The presence of multiple fractures is suspicious, as are old fractures in various stages of healing.
  - Look for human bite marks.
  - Look for head injuries – Level of consciousness, equal and reactive pupils, nausea/vomiting.
- ○ Older adults
  - Look for any bruises, lacerations, abrasions, or fractures in which the physical appearance does not match the history or mechanism of injury.

Collaborative Care

- Nursing Care
  - ○ All states have mandatory reporting laws that require nurses to report suspected abuse. There are civil and criminal penalties for not reporting suspicions of abuse.
  - ○ Nursing interventions for child or older adult abuse must include the following:
    - Mandatory reporting of suspected or actual cases of child or older adult abuse
    - Complete, accurate documentation of subjective and objective data obtained during data collection
  - ○ Conduct a nursing history.
    - Provide privacy when conducting interviews about family abuse.
    - Be direct, honest, and professional.
    - Use language the client understands.
    - Be understanding and attentive.
    - Use therapeutic techniques that demonstrate understanding.
    - Use open-ended questions to elicit descriptive responses.
    - Inform the client if a referral must be made to children's or adult protective services and explain the process.
  - ○ Provide basic care to treat injuries.
  - ○ Request appropriate referrals.

- o   Nursing interventions for rape
  - ■   Provide a private environment for an examination with a specially trained nurse-advocate, if available. A sexual assault nurse examiner (SANE) is a specially trained nurse who performs such examinations.
  - ■   Assist the specialist with the physical examination and the collection, documentation, and preservation of forensic evidence
  - ■   Provide nonjudgmental and empathetic care.
  - ■   Call the client's available personal support system, such as a partner or parents, if the client gives permission.
- o   Nursing interventions for community-wide or mass casualty incidents include:
  - ■   Early intervention
    - □   Provide psychological first aid:
      - ▸   Make sure clients are physically and psychologically safe from harm.
      - ▸   Reduce stress-related symptoms, such as using techniques to alleviate a panic attack.
      - ▸   Provide interventions to restore rest/sleep and meet other basic needs.
      - ▸   Provide links to social supports and information about critical resources.
    - □   Depending on their level of expertise and training, mental health nurses may provide assessment, consultation, therapeutic communication and support, triage, and psychological and physical care.
  - ■   Critical incident stress debriefing
    - □   This is a crisis intervention strategy used to assist individuals who have experienced a traumatic event, usually involving violence (staff experiencing client violence, school children and personnel experiencing the violent death of a student, rescue workers after an earthquake) in a safe environment.
    - □   Debriefing may take place in group meetings with a facilitator where thoughts and feelings may be expressed safely.
    - □   The facilitator will acknowledge reactions, provide anticipatory guidance for symptoms that may still occur, teach stress management techniques, and provide referrals.
    - □   The group may choose to meet on an ongoing basis or disband after resolution of the crisis.
- ●   Care After Discharge
  - o   Nursing actions
    - ■   Help client develop a safety plan, identify behaviors and situations that might trigger violence, and provide information regarding safe places to live.
    - ■   Encourage participation in support groups.

- - Use case management to coordinate community, medical, criminal justice, and social services.

  - Use crisis intervention techniques to help resolve family or community situations where violence has occurred.

  o Client education

  - Reinforce to clients self-care and empowerment skills.

  - Reinforce to clients ways to manage stress.

- Client Outcomes

  o The client will develop safety plan.

  o The client will participate in self-help or support group.

  o The client will identify strategies to manage stress.

  o The client will be free from injury.

Ⓐ APPLICATION EXERCISES

1. A nurse is caring for a client who has paranoid personality disorder. Which of the following statements made by the client is an example of aggressive communication? (Select all that apply.)

   _____ "I wish you would not make me angry."

   _____ "I feel angry when you leave me."

   _____ "It makes me angry when you interrupt me."

   _____ "You'd better listen to me."

   _____ "You are going to be punished for this."

2. A nurse is assisting with the admission of a client in an inpatient mental health unit. Which of the following findings should the nurse expect if the client is in the preassaultive stage of violence? (Select all that apply.)

   _____ Lethargy

   _____ Defensive responses to questions

   _____ Rapid breathing

   _____ Blunted affect

   _____ Loud, rapid talking

3. A nurse is preparing to administer medications to a client in an inpatient mental health setting. The client is playing cards with a group, and becomes angry and knocks the medications out of the nurse's hands. Which of the following is the priority nursing action?

   A. Encourage the client to express her feelings.

   B. Maintain eye contact with the client.

   C. Move the client away from others.

   D. Tell the client that the behavior is not acceptable.

4. A nurse is collecting data for a preschool-age child who was brought to the provider's office with reports of tenderness and bruising along the clavicle. Which of the following findings should the nurse consider suspicions of child abuse? (Select all that apply.)

   _____ Scabs on knees

   _____ Pinpoint burn marks on forearms

   _____ Appears passive

   _____ Mismatched clothing

   _____ Bruises on torso

5. A nurse is assisting with the care of a client who has been placed in seclusion. Which of the following statements about seclusion are correct? (Select all that apply.)

    _____ The nurse does not need a prescription to place the client in seclusion when the client's admission is involuntary.

    _____ The purpose of seclusion is to lead to positive behavior change.

    _____ The nurse should observe the client who is in seclusion at least every hour.

    _____ In some instances, intramuscular medications may be administered to calm the client.

    _____ The client has the right to request to be placed in seclusion.

APPLICATION EXERCISES ANSWER KEY

1. A nurse is caring for a client who has paranoid personality disorder. Which of the following statements made by the client is an example of aggressive communication? (Select all that apply.)

    _____ "I wish you would not make me angry."

    _____ "I feel angry when you leave me."

    _____ "It makes me angry when you interrupt me."

    __X__ **"You'd better listen to me."**

    __X__ **"You are going to be punished for this."**

    Using the words "You'd better" implies a threat (that something bad will happen if the person does not listen) and a lack of respect for the other individual. Telling the nurse that she will be punished for this also is threatening. The other options do not imply a threat.

    Ⓝ **NCLEX® Connection: Psychosocial Integrity, Therapeutic Communications**

2. A nurse is assisting with the admission of a client in an inpatient mental health unit. Which of the following findings should the nurse expect if the client is in the preassaultive stage of violence? (Select all that apply.)

    _____ Lethargy

    __X__ **Defensive responses to questions**

    __X__ **Rapid breathing**

    _____ Blunted affect

    __X__ **Loud, rapid talking**

    Defensive responses to questions, rapid breathing, and loud, rapid talking are findings that may indicate a client is in the preassaultive stage of violence. Lethargy and blunt affect are more likely to be found in a client who has depression.

    Ⓝ **NCLEX® Connection: Psychosocial Integrity, Mental Health Concepts**

3. A nurse is preparing to administer medications to a client in an inpatient mental health setting. The client is playing cards with a group, and becomes angry and knocks the medications out of the nurse's hands. Which of the following is the priority nursing action?

    A. Encourage the client to express her feelings.

    B. Maintain eye contact with the client.

    C. Move the client away from others.

    D. Tell the client that the behavior is not acceptable.

The greatest risk in the situation is harm to others. The priority action is for the nurse to move the client away from others to prevent injury. Encouraging the client to express feelings, maintaining eye contact with the client, and telling the client that her behavior is not acceptable are all important interventions, but they are not the priority.

Ⓝ **NCLEX® Connection: Psychosocial Integrity, Behavioral Interventions**

4. A nurse is collecting data for a preschool-age child who was brought to the provider's office with reports of tenderness and bruising along the clavicle. Which of the following findings should the nurse consider suspicions of child abuse? (Select all that apply.)

_____	Scabs on knees
__X__	**Pinpoint burn marks on forearms**
__X__	**Appears passive**
_____	Mismatched clothing
__X__	**Bruises on torso**

Pinpoint burn marks on the client's forearms may indicate burns caused by cigarettes, and bruises on the torso may indicate a beating. Children who are abused often appear passive and withdrawn. Scabs on the client's knees and mismatched clothing are expected findings in a preschool-age child, and are consistent with the child's developmental age.

Ⓝ **NCLEX® Connection: Psychosocial Integrity, Abuse or Neglect**

5. A nurse is assisting with the care of a client who has been placed in seclusion. Which of the following statements about seclusion are correct? (Select all that apply.)

_____ The nurse does not need a prescription to place the client in seclusion when the client's admission is involuntary.

_____ The purpose of seclusion is to lead to positive behavior change.

_____ The nurse should observe the client who is in seclusion at least every hour.

___X___ **In some instances, intramuscular medications may be administered to calm the client.**

___X___ **The client has the right to request to be placed in seclusion.**

Clients who are placed in seclusion may be administered intramuscular psychotropic medications. In some instances, the client may be placed in seclusion at the request of the client. In an emergency, the nurse may place the client in seclusion, but the nurse must obtain a verbal or written prescription from the provider as soon as possible for the seclusion, usually within 15 to 30 min. The purpose of seclusion is to protect the client from harming himself or others, and does not usually lead to a positive behavior change. The nurse should observe the client in seclusion at least every 15 min.

NCLEX® Connection: Safety and Infection Control, Restraints and Safety Devices

References

Hockenberry, M. J., & Wilson, D. (2009). *Wong's essentials of pediatric nursing* (8th ed.). St. Louis, MO: Mosby.

Lehne, R. A. (2010). *Pharmacology for nursing care* (7th ed.). St. Louis, MO: Saunders.

Roach, S. S., & Ford, S. M. (2008). *Introductory clinical pharmacology.* Philadelphia, PA: Lippincott Williams & Wilkins.

Townsend, M. C. (2008). *Essentials of psychiatric mental health nursing: Concepts of care in evidence-based practice* (4th ed.). Philadelphia, PA: F. A. Davis.

Varcarolis, E. M., Halter, M.J., (2010). *Foundations of psychiatric mental health nursing: A clinical approach* (6th ed.). St. Louis, MO: Saunders.

Wilson, B. A., Shannon, M. T., & Shields, K. M. (2011). *Pearson nurse's drug guide 2011.* Upper Saddle River, NJ: Pearson.